The 21-DAY SUGAR DETOX

THE FAST TRACK TO CRUSH CRAVINGS, LOSE WEIGHT FAST & FEEL BETTER NOW

The 21-DAY SUGAR DETOX

THE FAST TRACK TO CRUSH CRAVINGS, LOSE WEIGHT FAST & FEEL BETTER NOW

Cynthia A. Ray, MPH, RDN

DEDICATION

This book is dedicated to my husband, Corey, and our three children, Cooper, Camble, and Charlotte, for keeping our homeschooling life fulfilling and supporting me in my God-given desire to minister wellness education to our community.

SUGAR DETOX SUPPORT GROUP

Grab your spot in my Sugar Detox Online group. You will receive daily education, inspiration, coaching, and support from me and others on the same sugar-free journey.

Visit the link below to learn more:

www.21dayswithoutsugar.com

FOREWORD

The most powerful people on earth are those who have allowed God to turn their pain into purpose. And that's the secret to Cynthia Ray's success.

Having defeated the giant of food addiction in her own life, she's made it her mission to set other captives free. What I admire most about Cynthia is her commitment to excellence. Once she understood her calling, she pursued an advanced degree and multiple certifications to make sure she was offering the best of the best to those she felt called to serve.

It's one thing to have passion, it's quite another to develop mastery. After more than two decades as a registered dietitian and fitness expert, Cynthia knows exactly what it takes to help women break the bondage of sugar off of their lives.

In *The 21-Day Sugar Detox*, she's mapped out a well-balanced pathway to better health in spirit, soul and body. If you're looking for a faith-based approach to weight loss—one that will equip you with practical tools you can easily incorporate into your daily and weekly routine—then look no further. You've just found what you've been looking for!

Donna Partow,
Bestselling author,
Becoming the Woman I Want To Be: A 90-Day Journey to Renewing Spirit, Soul & Body

TABLE OF CONTENTS

INTRODUCTION

Welcome to the 21-Day Sugar Detox.

I am so happy you are here and have decided to take better care of yourself, physically and spiritually. It is so easy to fall into a pattern of excess sugar. I have been there too. Before you know it, you are habitually grabbing a sweet treat after dinner, a quick pick-me-up in the afternoon, or looking for chocolate when you feel stressed.

Maybe you're afraid you won't be able to stick with the program. You don't want to start and not finish. Well, I have great news for you. This program has been tested and it works every time, because I'm going to set you up for success. You may be surprised at how victorious you can be. Just follow along with the meal plan and daily devotionals one day at a time, and before you know it, the twenty-one days will be complete. You can do it!

This detox is different from anything you may have tried before, because we are going to invite the God of the universe to be with us every step of the way. You will strengthen spirit, soul and body. Get ready to see what God can in your life on this journey.

Each day of the twenty-one day detox, you will spend about ten to fifteen minutes reading the daily devotional, journaling, and praying. You will need about two hours at the end of each week for grocery shopping and meal planning. I recommend grocery shopping on Saturday morning and preparing meals and snacks on Sunday. Most days, what you prepare for dinner will be eaten for lunch the next day. The meals are basic and easy to follow, usually taking around 30-40 minutes to prepare.

I've included a wide variety of recipes at the back of the book. In addition, I've prepared free shopping lists and suggested meal plans, which you can download by visiting: www.21dayswithoutsugar.com

Plus I've built a supportive community online, so you never have to walk alone. Come join us and get the love and support you deserve. All the details are on the website listed above.

This program combines paleo-style eating and cleansing drinks—all carefully designed to balance your blood sugar, crush sugar cravings, reset your palate, banish belly fat, reduce inflammation, remove toxins, and refresh your body from the inside out so you can feel better now. And of course, you can expect to lose weight!

Before we get started, you should know that I don't blame every problem in your life on sugar. Nor do I declare it "evil" and forbidden forever. However, I have to be honest. If you don't feel on top of the world—physically and emotionally—chances are sugar plays a part. Sugar can affect your gut, energy level, immune system, teeth, weight, skin, sleep, and overall quality of life.

Sugar is not evil in itself, but the patterns it creates can cause you emotional and physical pain. Sugar may be where you run for emotional comfort. Or it's just a bad habit. Rest assured there will be plenty of grace here. If you fall into temptation and get off track, bring it to God—all of it: guilt, anxiety, anger, frustration, and your desire to throw in the towel. Lay it all at his feet and let his grace, peace, and truth wash over you.

Then start over.

Whether on-track or off-track, God's love for you is the same. Don't let your missteps sideline you. Keep your focus on the ultimate success you want in your life. Give your dreams to God, take a deep breath, and resolve that you *are* a successful person and success is the only option. If you have a bad day (or bad week!), pick up where you left off and keep going. I believe in you, and I pray you will choose to believe in yourself.

Quitting is not an option and not negotiable. It only takes approximately seven without sugar for cravings to diminish or even disappear. Keep going for twenty-one days to completely crush your cravings and develop new habits that will stick long-term.

In working with hundreds of clients and detoxing myself several times a year, I have found *everyone* has been able to reset their palate and kiss sugar cravings goodbye. It will be the same for you.

Post-cleanse, you will find you are sensitive to added sugars. The foods you ate before will taste too sweet for your new palate to enjoy. In other words, you can make permanent changes. This isn't a diet; it's a new way of living.

Do You Need a Sugar Detox?

How do you know whether or not the 21-Day Sugar Detox is right for you? Take a minute to read through the following signs and symptoms. Does any of this sound like you:

- Eat sweets even if you're not hungry?
- Experience sugar withdrawal symptoms?
- Suspect that you might have an issue with drug or alcohol abuse?

- Have a family history of drug or alcohol abuse?
- Get out of bed at night to eat sweets?
- Have skin eruptions/breakouts?
- Experience constant fatigue?
- Find yourself hiding your sugar habit?
- Have headaches?
- Not sleeping well and waking up nauseous?
- Have tooth decay or cavities?
- Feeling hungry even though you just ate?
- Get bloated after you eat?
- Feel shame and guilt when you eat sugar?
- Have an all-or-nothing relationship with sugar?

If you answered yes to three or more, guess what? You need *The 21-Day Sugar Detox*! You have the right book in your hands at the right time. This is your moment, friend. You are now on the fast track to crush cravings, lose weight fast, and feel better now. I'm so excited for you.

All of these issues are about to get resolved. Follow along each day in this book, and I will show you exactly what to eat and how to start your day to ensure success. I also will give you daily tips and supplement recommendations to improve your overall health.

My Story

In my young adult years, I struggled with a chaotic and dysfunctional relationship with food and my body image. I learned that our culture says "thin and fit are beautiful." So I was determined to be slim and healthy.

I played soccer and softball from age five until age eighteen. I loved competition and the satisfaction of beating my opponent. I also enjoyed testing my body and pushing it to the limit to see what it could do.

During my first year of college—away from home for the first time—I was depressed and suffered from deep feelings of abandonment. I developed an insatiable urge to eat sugar. I would search through the pantry at the home I shared with my sorority sisters and look for something to bake or rush to the grocery store for a half-gallon of fat-free ice cream. I'd devour almost all of it on my own.

These urges became a regular thing for me. They sank into my emotions, and the guilt became unbearable. One night while in the middle of a binge, something triggered in my mind.

The thought that I could enjoy as much as I wanted without the calories was an ingenious idea. Binging on my favorite forbidden food followed by vomiting felt good the first time, and I was excited to make this discovery. Soon, I was in a battle with bulimia and an endless cycle of binging and purging–induced vomiting and excessive exercise.

The glands in my neck were swollen, my eyes were bloodshot, and my face was bloated. I was lightheaded, my body hurt, and I was always tired.

One night during my sophomore year, after purging, I looked into the bathroom mirror and got a real glimpse of my face. My eyes were red and watery, my skin was pale, and my spirit was empty. My face looked deformed and almost evil. I cried and felt the comfort of the Lord around me.

I needed this to end. And I was ready to get help.

While still in college I ended up in a twelve-month treatment program for eating disorders. The ladies in the program were all shapes and sizes. There were overeaters, under-eaters, bulimics, and chronic dieters. I learned that despite being different sizes, we all had the same struggle.

Recovery was a bumpy road, and I spent time in and out of the hospital. But finally, I was set free through much prayer and the power of the Holy Spirit.

That was more than twenty years ago. I thank God I have remained free from a dysfunctional relationship with food. In my two decades of private practice as a dietitian, I have been blessed to help many men and women get free from bondage to food– in particular, their addiction to sugar.

Now It's Your Turn

I will walk you into the same freedom, using the same tools I share with my coaching clients. You may or may not have had the same past as mine, but we are the same. You and I have struggled with something that feels bigger than us. And we desire the freedom to live without being a slave to sugar.

How the 21-Day Sugar Detox Works

Did you know toxins can be introduced to your body through environmental pollutants, the chemicals in foods you eat, refined sugars, alcohol, nicotine, illegal drugs, food preservatives, pesticides, prescription drugs, dental procedures, lotions, and soaps.

Our bodies store toxins within fat cells, which causes them to increase in size. Toxins are fat soluble, meaning they need fats to be sustained. To be flushed, they have to be converted to water-soluble by the liver. Through a complex series of processes, toxins can be eliminated by sweat, urine, and feces.

You can eliminate toxins and lose weight by eating lots of healthy veggies and whole foods. When you detoxify, you release toxins from fat cells and shrink them. And who doesn't want to shrink fat cells?

Here is the strategy:

1. Each daily reading will include an opportunity for reflection, key points to remember, ways to put the teaching into practice. I've even included a short prayer and affirmation for you to recite.

2. Eliminate refined sugar and alcoholic beverages for twenty-one days.

3. Eat according to the meal plan. (Recipes at the back of the book; a free sample meal plan is available at www.21dayswithoutsugar.com)

4. Enjoy cleansing juices and detox teas for an extra boost.

5. Refuse to be discouraged or intimidated by sugar withdrawal symptoms. They typically only last a few days.

6. You can do this program alone, but I encourage you to work through it with a group, either online or in your local community.

Be Alert to Detox Symptoms

Okay, I've shared lots of great news and encouragement so far. But now, I have to warn you about something. Before you feel better… you will probably *feel worse*. But I promise it won't last! Take a moment, right now, to mentally prepare yourself. That way, if you feel sick in the beginning, you won't panic. You'll know that it's all perfectly normal. You are just experiencing the usual detox symptoms. These symptoms[1] can include:

- Intense cravings for sugar.
- Headaches.
- Irritability.
- Fatigue.
- Muscle aches.
- Nausea, bloating, or other gastrointestinal issues.
- Anxiety or depression.
- Skin eruptions or breakouts.

This may sound hard to believe, but detox symptoms are actually something to celebrate. Yes, celebrate! It means the program is working and your body is healing. Isn't that wonderful? Spend extra time in prayer, thanking God for the work he is doing in purifying your body and making you whole.

What We'll Accomplish Together

So let's summarize what we can expect to accomplish together by the end of the twenty-one days. You will:

- Lose weight.
- Feel energized.

---

[1] Notice that detox symptoms do not include a fever. If you are experiencing a fever, please contact your local health care practitioner.

- Crave healthier foods.
- Stabilize your blood sugar.
- Get better sleep.
- Enjoy healthier skin.
- Eliminate bloating.
- Strengthen your immune system.
- Get rid of headaches.
- Heal more quickly when you do get sick.

All of that, just by changing what you put in your mouth.

Remember, this isn't a fad diet and it's not a crash diet. It's a healing protocol strategically designed to help your body *stop craving harmful foods* and *start craving healthy foods*. Won't it be amazing when your body becomes *your ally* as you move closer to becoming the woman you've always dreamed you could be? Goodbye yo-yo dieting. Goodbye self-sabotage. You are twenty-one days away from a brand new you.

I've seen God work miracles through this program with my coaching clients and I can't wait to hear *your* testimony someday soon.

Turn to Day 1 and let's get started!

THE JOURNEY TO FREEDOM

"I have the right to do anything" you say—but
not everything is beneficial. "I have the right to do
anything"—but I will not be mastered by anything.

—1 Corinthians 6:12

Welcome to Day 1. Take time to scan the table of contents to get an idea of what you will learn over the next twenty-one days. You can also turn to the back to review the recipes. If you want everything mapped out for you, be sure to grab the suggested weekly meal plan (including grocery lists) at www.21dayswithoutsugar. com.

Your success is based on advance preparation, commitment, and desire to get this done. I will get into the details on Day 2. Starting today, you should carry a water bottle wherever you go. Drink *lots* of water *(at least thirty-two ounces three times per day)* to flush out toxins.

If you don't already have a special place where you have quiet time in the morning, choose a place and make it pretty. Maybe buy some colorful pens or a small bouquet of flowers. Make it somewhere you'll look forward to sitting at the start of your day.

During the first few days, prepare in advance for when sugar cravings strike. Ensure you have the right foods handy to avoid the pattern of turning to carbs whenever you let yourself get too hungry.

Reflect

What's wrong with sugar?

Research has consistently connected regular sugar consumption with chronic internal inflammation, which can have profound long-term health implications—bowel diseases such as Crohn's, irritable bowel syndrome, diverticulitis, and Type 2 diabetes. Regular sugar consumption will cause bloating after meals, headaches, constant hunger, tooth decay, chronic illness, chronic fatigue, gut imbalance, fungal overgrowth, and poor skin health.

Eating sugar satisfies a craving but also causes an overgrowth of candida and yeast in your gut. This can cause brain fog, rashes, digestive issues, and a weakened immune system.

Not only does sugar negatively affect your gut health, but it worsens internal inflammation, which is a redness and swelling inside your body similar to what occurs outside your body when bitten by a bug. Internal inflammation is the cause of acute and chronic illnesses such as migraines, poor digestion, constipation, diabetes, leaky gut, heart disease, hormonal imbalances, chronic sickness, and allergies.

Living on a paleo-style diet for the next twenty-one days will set you up for total detox. It also will balance your hormones to control appetite and help you lose weight, without ever feeling deprived.

The best part is that you will balance your blood sugar and reduce sugar cravings.

Kicking sugar can be a struggle. Knowing how harmful sugar is can motivate you. When you are free from cravings, you'll feel light, healthy, and energized, with clear and radiant skin.

Many have gotten stuck in the "sugar cycle," also called the Carb Addiction Cycle, and struggle to get out. It can become an endless loop of cravings and low blood sugar unless you learn to take a detour.

The Carb Addiction Cycle begins with cravings caused by low blood sugar. Here is how it works:

Low Blood Sugar —> Cravings —>Eat Carbs —>High Blood Sugar —> Insulin Release —>Body Fat Production —-> Low Blood Sugar

A sugar craving is your body's way of telling you something. Your body gives you a lot of signals every day. However, these signals can be very subtle, so it's easy to ignore them.

While it's easier for some people to overcome cravings, others might have difficulty. We must understand the root of the problem. Emotions, hormone imbalance, addictive properties in the food, spiritual issues, or dietary imbalances can cause a craving.

Combat Cravings

Use this list to combat cravings:

- Use your cravings as a cue to stop and pray.
- Take ten deep belly breaths to release any tension.

- Exercise daily. Make it a combination of three days a week of strength exercise, three days a week of 20-30 minutes of cardio and one day of rest or stretching.

- Go outside and get fresh air.

- Organize something—purse, wallet, drawer, closet, car, desk.

- Grab a hot beverage, such as unsweetened tea, unsweetened coffee, or the cleanse tea listed on the meal plan.

- Brush your teeth.

- Chew sugar-free gum.

- Take a hot shower or warm bath for 5-10 minutes.

- Call a friend.

- Take magnesium, phosphorus, or sulfur.

- Take 500mg of L-Glutamine three times a day and an extra dose when you get a strong desire for something sweet. Try a quarter of a teaspoon, or open a 500mg capsule of L-Glutamine, place it under your tongue whenever you get a craving.

- Enjoy and savor two small squares of 85 percent dark chocolate or a cup of coffee or tea.

- Sit, breathe, and mediate. I like

  https://thechristianmeditator.com or the Abide app or YouTube channel https://www.youtube.com/c/AbideChristianMeditation.

Keep these tips in mind during your twenty-one day detox:

- Plan meals and snacks in advance before heading to the grocery store.

- Scan your meal plan for the day and keep it on hand for reference. Take a screenshot of it on your phone, print it out, or access it in your email inbox from your phone.

- Take food with you when you leave the house, in case you get hungry.
- Combine protein with fat to balance your blood sugar.

Kicking the sugar habit isn't all that complex. It's simple but not always easy, which is why we are on this journey together. With support and accountability, the hard stuff is challenging but doable.

Key Points

- Sugar causes conditions such as tooth decay, weight gain, candida, decreased energy, poor sleep, joint pain, and internal inflammation.
- Detoxing from sugar reduces internal inflammation, decreases your risk for illness, and can even reduce chronic health issues.
- The Carb Addiction Cycle can become an endless loop of cravings and low blood sugar unless you learn to take a detour.

Put it Into Practice

- Follow Day 1 of the meal plan (www.21dayswithoutsugar. com) and eliminate sugar and alternative sweeteners, including Xylitol, Erythritol, and Stevia. Know you cannot kick a sugar addiction while eating sugar alternatives. I will explain more in Day 12.
- Know you are in control, and you can choose to say no.

Prayer

Lord, forgive me as I forgive myself for the guilt, shame, and anxiety I allowed sugar to give me. I know everything is permissible for me, but not everything is beneficial. Your Word says, "Everything is permissible for me— but I will not be mastered by anything" (1 Corinthians 6:12). I do not want to be mastered by anything or anyone but you. I dedicate this cleanse to you for your glory and the health of my body. Please give me the strength and courage I need to get through these twenty-one days. Please help me to conquer this giant and come out victorious. I can do this with you and am excited to feel invigorated, alive, and well. Amen.

Affirmation

Write down the following affirmation, take a deep breath, clear any negative thoughts, say it out loud *three* times, and allow it to sink deep into your heart:

"I can say no to sugar, and I will be okay.
I am not mastered by anything but by God.
Today is my Day 1."

Checkup

Day 1 is done. Celebrate your success. Journal your thoughts and prayers.

CLEAN SUGAR OUT OF YOUR KITCHEN

Do you not know that your bodies are temples of the
Holy Spirit, who is in you, whom you have received
from God? You are not your own; you were bought at a
price. Therefore honor God with your bodies.

—1 Corinthians 6:19-20

Reflect

One of the critical keys to losing sugar cravings is to keep your blood sugar in check by eating regular, nutritionally balanced meals. Avoid getting too hungry. Eat often, if need be, and stick to the daily meal plan. And get rid of tempting sugar in your home.

This quick list of foods to remove will help you on your twenty-one-day journey.

Remove These Foods

Foods with added sugars, refined wheat, alcohol, soy, dairy (milk, butter, cheese, sour cream, yogurt), white potatoes, white rice, artificial sweeteners, dried fruit, artificial colors and flavorings, fast and processed foods, gluten-free grains, fruit juices, cured deli meats, and cured bacon, processed foods, grains (wheat, cereal, bread, oats, pasta, rice, barley, rye).

Keep These Foods

Meats (especially grass-fed or pasture-raised), grass-fed dairy, plain unsweetened coconut milk yogurt, almond milk, almond butter, non-starchy vegetables (broccoli, leafy greens, bell peppers, sea vegetables, asparagus), coffee and tea, nuts and seeds, fish and shellfish (preferably wild-caught, Omega-3 rich), eggs, starchy vegetables (butternut squash, sweet potatoes, carrots, beets), fermented vegetables (sauerkraut, kimchi, Lacto-fermented pickles), quinoa, healthy fats (avocado and olives), some fruit (one serving, sometimes two as listed in the meal plan).

Clean Out

Eliminate self-sabotage by removing everything from your kitchen that contains added sugar. That includes your pantry, fridge, and freezer. Give it away or throw it away.

Put it Into Practice

Now that you have taken sugar out of your home, it's time to plan and prepare for the weeks ahead. We are busy people with many distractions in our lives—family outings, sports activities, and spur-of-the-moment schedule surprises. Planning is key.

Plan meals for the week. I have found that Saturday works best for me. Look at the meal plan for the week and make your grocery list. These planning tips might help:

1. Plan to make your grocery list and shop on the weekend.

2. Make sure you are fed and hydrated before you shop.

3. Shop online for your groceries at your local market for a more convenient option.

Prayer

Lord, I know that my kitchen doesn't always have the healthiest foods, but I am ready and committed to eliminating what is harmful to my health and replacing it with healthy, life-giving foods. Help me stay consistent with meal planning for the week, so I can live out the outcome of this cleanse I so desire. Amen.

Affirmation

Write down the following affirmation, take a deep breath, clear any negative thoughts, say it out loud *three* times, and allow it to sink deep into your heart:

> "I keep only whole foods with no added sugar in my kitchen and shop for groceries on Saturday."

Checkup

No need to share what you are doing with the world. Let your results be the proof. Journal your experiences so far.

CLEANSE SUPPLEMENTS

No temptation has overtaken you except what is
common to mankind. And God is faithful; he will not
let you be tempted beyond what you can bear.
But when you are tempted, he will also provide a way
out so that you can endure it.

—1 Corinthians 10:13

Reflect

Glutathione is made up of the amino acids found in surprisingly high levels in most cells. It is especially concentrated in the liver, which plays a significant role in detoxification. Within the liver, glutathione binds to toxic molecules to prepare them for removal from the body.

Glutathione is the second-most abundant molecule in the body, just behind water. A family of enzymes called glutathione S-transferases (GSTs) is responsible for binding glutathione to these toxins, including excess hormones, man-made chemicals, environmental pollutants, pharmaceuticals, and heavy metals, preparing them for excretion. Glutathione helps make the toxins water-soluble so they can easily be flushed from your body. Glutathione not only works as a detoxifier but also an antioxidant.

Unfortunately, taking glutathione in a pill form does not absorb well. However, taking Gamma-Glutamylcysteine (GGC) will stimulate your body to produce more glutathione and keep levels elevated. A company called "Continual G" created a supplemental form of GGC called "Glyteine."

My family and I take it daily. I highly recommend adding this "master antioxidant" to your daily regimen to prevent illness and disease, as well as promote enhanced detoxification of sugars and other toxins your body is exposed to.

Within the first few weeks, you'll notice your body will eliminate toxins through your skin, urine, feces, sweat, or some combination of those. You may notice skin eruptions (acne or rash) or a smell from your sweat, urine, or feces. Don't worry. This is temporary and is a good sign the toxins are leaving your liver. At the same time, your body is getting energized and reversing the aging process.

Glutathione is known for heavy metal liver detoxification. As a result, you will heal more quickly from injuries, experience faster recovery from illness, recover from exercise-induced soreness more quickly, and see clearer, glowing skin.

We can experience decreased levels of glutathione and not even know it. This list includes the most common reasons for the limited production of glutathione:

- Aging
- Illness
- Strenuous exercise

- Unhealthy lifestyle choices
- Environmental toxins and pollutants
- Medications
- Stress
- Poor diet

A few of my favorite supplements for detoxing sugar include:

- Iron and Riboflavin
- Vitamins A, C, E, K, B1, and B6
- Goldenseal, echinacea, grape seed, dandelion, schizandra, milk thistle, garlic, rosemary, and poke root.
- Minerals copper, selenium, and zinc.
- A probiotic.

If you have any of these at home already, you can add the others to your daily cleansing regimen. The amount you need will be listed on the bottle.

Key Points

- Discover glutathione, herbs, vitamins, and minerals that help your liver and immune system during the detox process.
- Head to your local health food store or go online and pick up glutathione (Glyteine), a probiotic, a high-quality multivitamin, or herbal remedy of choice from the list above.

Put it Into Practice

Go online, head to the store, take a look in your home and grab one or two of the listed supplements to aid your body in ridding the body of toxins, especially if you have detox symptoms. Having these supplements on hand will help speed up the process and ensure all toxins are completely removed.

Prayer

Thank you, Lord, for the food in nature and for giving me an understanding of what my body needs more of instead of the sugar that I used to crave. I want to desire the foods that fulfill all my physical needs. Amen.

Affirmation

Write down the following affirmation, take a deep breath, clear any negative thoughts, say it out loud *three* times, and allow it to sink deep into your heart:

> "I eat a balanced diet making sure to supplement with additional nutrients to give my body all it needs to function optimally."

Checkup

You are just getting started. Take a moment to self-assess. On a scale of 1-10, how would you rate your progress through the first three days?

FOODS THAT SATISFY SUGAR CRAVINGS

So whether you eat or drink or whatever you do, do it
all for the glory of God.

—1 Corinthians 10:31

Reflect

Today's Bible verse reminds us that what you choose to eat and drink should also be done for God's glory. It shows us that living with godly character includes day-to-day things like eating and drinking.

In 1 Corinthians 10:23, God reminds us that we have free will, but he stands ready to guide us into the right choices: "I have the right to do anything," you say—but not everything is beneficial. "I have the right to do anything"—but not everything is constructive.

You can choose to eat whatever you want, but it may not always feel as good in your body as the idea seemed in your mind. How often have you chosen to eat a sugary treat because it "felt" like a good idea but regretted it later because you didn't feel well?

For many of us, urges for chocolate or sugary foods creep in at certain times of the month. Perhaps you are angry, lonely, tired, overwhelmed, frustrated, etc., and can't get your mind off something sweet to soothe your emotions.

About eight years ago, when I first started cleansing, I noticed cravings kicked in after three to five days of not having sugar. I thought of brownies and ice cream all the time. If I wasn't thinking about either, I saw commercials on TV or the Internet or ads in magazines for chocolate.

I searched for whatever I could get my hands on as a sugar alternative to satisfy my cravings, including recipes that contained no refined sugar or artificial sweeteners. I was excited when I discovered 85 percent dark chocolate and no-sugar-added sunflower seed butter. Both of those options satisfied my craving and saved me from slipping up.

Every time I cleansed, the cravings became less and less. Eventually, I discovered I could be okay with coffee, a small piece of 85 percent dark chocolate, flavored sparkling water, and some fruit with nut butter.

In addition to a well-balanced diet with plenty of protein, this list of supplements will help alleviate sugar cravings. They are also great for helping you sleep better and regulate hormones. Take the amount recommended on the bottle for a daily serving.

Magnesium
A magnesium deficiency could be the cause of your chocolate cravings. Naturally occurring in whole grains, nuts, spinach, and grains, the recommended daily amount is 400mg. Taking a supplement

while on a detox can keep your cravings in check. As an added benefit, magnesium also can give you a great night's sleep.

L-Glutamine

L-Glutamine is an amino acid converted into a neurotransmitter that helps curb sugar cravings. Researchers have found that L-glutamine plays a role in diminishing normal sugar cravings.

For instance, when blood sugar is low, glutamine quickly and easily converts to a pure form of glucose, having no effect on insulin levels and keeping blood sugar levels stable. Taking L-Glutamine can help avoid reaching for high-sugar foods such as candy, cookies, and cakes.

As mentioned earlier, taking 500mg three times a day and an extra dose when you get a strong desire for something sweet.

Vitamin D

If Vitamin D gets depleted, leptin levels decrease, causing you to feel hungry. Leptin is the hormone that helps to turn off your appetite. If you don't have enough Vitamin D, you constantly may feel hungry. Your body naturally gets this vitamin from sunshine, but it's best to supplement in regions with less sun. Foods with naturally-occurring Vitamin D include eggs and fish.

Omega-3 Fatty Acids

Omega-3 regulates normal brain function, which controls mood and reduces sugar cravings by balancing blood sugar.

Chromium picolinate

Taking this supplement will help to regulate blood sugar levels. Your body uses blood sugar as fuel and reduces cravings. Chromium is in broccoli, beans, pork chops, turkey, hazelnuts, and asparagus.

Zinc

Zinc helps with blood sugar and hormone response. A zinc deficiency can be another cause of cravings for something sweet. Zinc is found naturally in beef, lamb, chicken, turkey, eggs, and chickpeas.

Vitamin B

Vitamin B can help with carbohydrate metabolism. Your body may experience further cravings because it is naturally trying to get B vitamins from ingesting carbohydrates. Vitamin B6 can be found in beef, chicken, turkey, tuna, avocado, sunflower seeds, and sesame seeds.

Phosphorus and sulfur also are great for calming the body and sugar cravings.

Eating a sugary treat can trigger cravings for the next few days. When this happens to me, I use my sweet treat alternatives to reset my palate and take the desires away with whole, satisfying, nutritious foods. You can learn more at: www.wellwithinutrition. com/10-sweet-treat-alternatives

Key Points

- Use the sweet treat alternatives list to reset your palate.
- You may be deficient in a number of nutrients, and that's what's causing your sugar cravings. Eating a well-balanced diet of healthy meats, fish, veggies, and supplementation can help.

Put it Into Practice

You don't have to mourn the loss of sugar and feel sorry for yourself. Instead, find foods that will satisfy your cravings and heal your body. Choose at least one or two of the supplements listed. Buy from your local health food store or place an order on Amazon to have something on hand to help curb cravings.

Prayer

Lord, help me to remember the foods that glorify you as I make healthier choices. Thank you for the wisdom shared here and for making it easier for me to glorify you with the foods I choose to eat. Amen.

Affirmation

Write down the following affirmation, take a deep breath, clear any negative thoughts, say it out loud *three* times, and allow it to sink deep into your heart:

> "I've got this and can enjoy sweet treat alternatives as my palate adjusts."

Checkup

You are about to pass through to the other side where cravings will be gone. Remember, when things get more challenging, they are just about to get easier.

There's no going back now. How do you feel compared to how you felt on Day 4?

CLEANSING FOODS

Blessed are You, Lord our God, Ruler of the universe,
who creates the fruit of the tree.
Blessed are You, Lord our God, Ruler of the universe,
who creates the fruit of the ground.

—Jewish Blessing for Food and Drink

Reflect

Being in nature is my happy place. A few years ago, my husband and I took a guided hike in Maui. Along the way, I stumbled upon roots of ginger growing in the middle of the trail. I had never seen anything like it before. Every flower was exotic and perfect. So perfect that I questioned whether or not they were real. They were. I dug up the ginger roots and picked the lush, brightly colored tropical fruits hanging above.

The following spring, when the kids were in elementary school, I took them to a local family-owned farm for a homeschool group field trip. We all hopped onto a large wagon pulled by a farm tractor for a tour. At the end of our time, the driver allowed us to hop out and pick whatever produce we wanted from acres of crops. We went through rows and rows of green onions, carrots, lettuce, tomatoes of all sizes and shapes, squash, eggplant, beets, cilantro, and peas. We had so much fun roaming through the rows and getting our hands dirty. The fragrant smell of growing cilantro in the air was intoxicating.

As soon as we got home, we filled buckets with water and swished our freshly picked produce to remove the excess dirt before storing and juicing. The kids chose celery, carrots, cilantro, beet, and apple for juicing. After all of that hard work, the luscious taste of fresh juice was so refreshing. Since fresh produce is packed with vitamins, minerals, water, and fiber, they are naturally cleansing and perfect for our bodies. However, a handful of foods pack an even bigger punch for liver, gut, and total body toxin cleansing–ginger, celery, beets, lemon, cabbage, spinach, broccoli, kale, parsley, lettuce greens, cilantro, sweet potatoes, cauliflower, and cucumber.

These foods are filled with vitamins and antioxidants that help your body's natural ability to cleanse and detoxify itself, remove toxins, and give you the necessary nutrients to lead a happy and healthy life.

Top Veggies to Juice For Detoxification

- Cucumber: It's 95 percent water and is an incredible detoxifier, helping with liver and kidney function.

- Lemon: Is one of the essential items to stock in your kitchen and is an effective cleansing agent.

- Beets: Contain nutrients that may help lower your blood pressure, fight inflammation, and support detoxification.[2]

______

[2] McKay Gorse, "9 Foods to Naturally Detox," Health Matters, February 26, 2019, patientfirst.com/blog/9-foods-to-naturally-detox

Two of my favorite detox juice recipes are[3]:

Ultimate Green Detox Juice

Ingredients

- 2 green apples cut in half
- 3 stalks of celery with no leaves
- 1 cucumber
- 8 leaves of kale
- 1/2 lemon peeled
- 1 piece of fresh ginger
- Sprig of mint (optional)
- 1 beet

Instructions

1. Wash all the ingredients well and pat dry.
2. Cut fruit and vegetables into 1-2 inch chunks. Remove any peels.
3. Place all ingredients in a juicer. If you don't have a juicer, you can use a blender and use a fine strainer to remove the solid portions.
4. Process into juice according to the manufacturer's directions.

---

[3] Audrey Johns, "10 Detox Juice Recipes for Weight Loss Cleanse | Juice Cleanse," Lose Weight by Eating, Celebrating Healthy Recipes, 2022, https://loseweightbyeating.com/10-detox-juice-recipes-weight-loss-cleanse/

Green Ginger Ale Weight Loss Juice

Ingredients

- 1 medium apple
- 4 stalks of celery
- 2 cups of spinach
- 2 cucumbers
- 1 piece of ginger root one-inch long
- 1 lime peeled

Instructions

1. Wash all the ingredients well and pat dry.
2. Cut fruit and vegetables into 1-2 inch chunks. Remove any peels.
3. Place all of the ingredients in a juicer. If you don't have a juicer, you can use a blender and use a fine strainer to remove the solid portions.
4. Process into juice according to the manufacturer's directions.

Key Points

The top benefits of cleansing juices:

1. Helps you lose weight quickly.
2. Improves nutrient absorption.
3. Feeds good bacteria in your gut.
4. Helps lower cholesterol.
5. Helps detox your liver.
6. Lowers blood sugar levels.

7. Improves your skin.

8. Broadens the range of vegetables you eat.

Put it Into Practice

Use the meal plan to include cleansing foods and juices each day to help your body in the cleansing process. You can download the meal plan at www.21dayswithoutsugar.com.

Prayer

Lord, Thank you for the natural food that serves to assist in cleansing my body of toxins. Lord, you are great, and I look forward to living the long and healthy life you have set before me. Amen.

Affirmation

Write down the following affirmation, take a deep breath, clear any negative thoughts, say it out loud *three* times, and allow it to sink deep into your heart:

"I will eat lots of colorful produce."

Checkup

Celebrate you, every bit of you, and your power to overcome. What can you applaud?

CLEANSING DRINK

Nevertheless, I will bring health and healing to it;
I will heal my people and will let them enjoy abundant
peace and security.

—Jeremiah 33:6

Reflect

Have you ever awakened with a gnawing feeling in your stomach? A sense of being nauseous and super hungry simultaneously?

For years I thought I was super hungry. And although I ate something, I continued to feel slightly nauseous for the rest of the day.

After some time, I discovered that feelings of nausea in the morning were usually the result of a late-night snack, dessert, alcoholic beverage, or large meal. When I made this discovery, I understood the nausea was caused by undigested food sitting in my stomach for hours.

I wasn't hungry. I needed a way to soothe my nausea.

When you feel this way, avoid eating carbohydrate-rich foods, which increase stomach acidity. Instead, eat alkaline-producing foods, such as lemon, to neutralize it.

I searched for a cleansing drink recipe to alleviate my nausea. In my search, I discovered my favorite "go-to" body cleansing, anti-inflammatory, and stomach acid-neutralizing drink recipe. I use this recipe when I detox from sugar, need cleansing after vacation, a holiday, or a celebration meal, or find myself eating closer to bedtime than I'd like. I'm including it below.

The list includes:

- Apple cider vinegar: Naturally balances your body's pH and blood sugar levels. It contains a number of enzymes and acts as a probiotic and improves gut health. It also helps in detoxing the liver and lymphatic system.

- Lemon: Is known for its cleansing properties and ability to help with weight loss. It is high in minerals and has multiple vitamins such as Vitamin C and folate, which help balance your pH and nourish your body.

- Raw honey: Is great for boosting your immune system. It has enzymes, vitamins, and minerals that nourish the body while you detox.

- Fresh ginger: Is a remedy for digestive issues and will give your gut a substantial health boost with its anti-inflammatory properties.

- Cayenne pepper: Is a natural fat burner with anti-inflammatory effects and will help detoxify your body.

Yes, the recipe below is spicy. Sip on it and swirl it around with each sip since the ingredients settle. You will feel better in no time.

Apple Cider Vinegar Detox Recipe

- 1 cup water
- 2 tablespoons apple cider vinegar
- 2 tablespoons of freshly squeezed lemon juice
- 1 teaspoon fresh ginger or ground ginger
- ¼ teaspoon ground cinnamon
- 1 dash of cayenne pepper
- ½ teaspoon of honey (optional if the drink is too strong at first)

Key Point

- Be sure to enjoy a cleansing drink each day.

Put it Into Practice

Enjoy this cleansing drink to boost your detox, reduce inflammation in your body, and feel refreshed.

Prayer

Thank you, Lord, for giving us herbs and plants on the earth to help our bodies heal and recover. I want to care for my body and honor you in the process. I pray the plants in this drink will bless my body and bring the cleansing it needs. Amen.

Affirmation

Write down the following affirmation, take a deep breath, clear any negative thoughts, say it out loud three times, and allow it to sink deep into your heart:

"I commit to you having all the ingredients on hand so I can enjoy them

when I need them. I will use a soothing beverage to feel refreshed from the inside out."

Checkup

You might be just getting over the hump of the full detox time. Keep going. The detox will get easier from here. What's your biggest takeaway so far?

____

____

____

____

NATURAL DIURETIC

Those who cleanse themselves from the latter will be instruments for special purposes, made holy, useful to the Master and prepared to do any good work.

—2 Timothy 2:21

Reflect

Eating a diet with lots of carbs and sugar can cause water retention and puffiness throughout your body. My answer for water retention relief is hot lemon water. Not only does it release extra water, but it also cleanses you.

When I was pregnant with my daughter, I retained a lot of water. My face was puffy, and my ankles were swollen. Because I was pregnant, I couldn't take a diuretic, which is "any substance that increases urination, helping flush water from your system."[4] I went online to see if I could find a natural form that I could try.

---

[4] Jody Braverman, CPT, FNS, RYT, "Is Lemon a Natural Diuretic," LiveStrong.Com, 2022, https://www.livestrong.com/article/16266-lemon-natural-diuretic/

I discovered lemons steeped in hot water pull excess water out of your body and excrete it through your urine. I followed the recipe and sipped on my newfound drink. In the article, the writer also recommended I drink it before bed so it could flush out fluids and toxins overnight. The drink worked quickly, and my swelling decreased noticeably.

To this day, I like to keep lemons on hand, just in case I need a little boost. The mixture is great for cleansing and an excellent stomach acid neutralizer. This miracle recipe can be found in your meal plan.

Hot Lemon Water

Ingredients

- 1-2 lemons
- 2-3 cups of water

Directions

1. Slice lemons in half and squeeze juice from the slices into a pan with water.
2. Bring water to a boil. Reduce to a simmer for five minutes.
3. Remove from heat and let cool for five minutes.
4. Add a little cool water if you are short on time and need it to cool more quickly. Pour the water into a mug with one of the lemons from your pan. Doing this will allow the lemon to continue steeping while you drink it.

Also, drink hot lemon water near bedtime. You'll sleep better and wake up feeling refreshed.

A few additional health benefits of drinking hot lemon water include:

- Boosts the immune system.
- Balances pH in the body.
- Helps reduce hunger and supports weight loss.
- Aids digestion and provides nutrients.
- Improves urinary health—acts as a gentle, natural diuretic.
- Creates clear, glowing skin.
- Hydrates the lymph system and supports adrenals.

One potential drawback, however, is the citric acid in lemon juice could erode the enamel on your teeth. Ensure the water is lukewarm and not steaming hot to prevent damage.

Make sure to wait sixty minutes after drinking to brush your teeth to avoid scrubbing the citric acid into your teeth.

Key Point

- Hot lemon water reduces water retention, alleviates an acidic stomach, and cleanses your whole body.

Put it Into Practice

Drink a cup of hot lemon water before bed. It's a natural alternative for diuretics to rid excess water and toxins.

Make sure to head to the grocery store if you didn't yesterday and get ready for week two.

Prayer

Thank you, Lord, for plant foods such as lemons that seem so simple but can be beneficial to cleanse my body. Amen.

Affirmation

Write down the following affirmation, take a deep breath, clear any negative thoughts, say it out loud *three* times, and allow it to sink deep into your heart:

> "Hot lemon water is the drink I go to first when I feel like I'm retaining water."

Checkup

How do you feel? Write down something that surprised you about yourself on this journey so far.

STAY HYDRATED

But whoever drinks the water I give them will never thirst. Indeed, the water I give them will become in them a spring of water welling up to eternal life.

—John 4:14

Reflect

About a year ago, I noticed in pictures that my face and arms looked puffy. I thought I was fat or maybe just had gained more muscle from my workout program. I didn't like how I looked but ignored the appearance because the pictures didn't match how fit and firm I was in real life.

Fast forward to a year later, I came across a YouTube video of a young woman who had done a seven-day, one-gallon water hydration challenge. I knew I was not drinking enough water. At that point, my skin was breaking out and my eyes were dry. I thought maybe underhydration was the problem. I bought myself a thirty-four ounce water bottle. I had to drink four bottles to get in the entire gallon daily.

At the end of the seven days, I created a new habit and took my water bottle with me wherever I went. This new habit has stuck with me ever since, although I don't drink an entire gallon every day, I certainly drink plenty.

Adding additional water to your day will initially cause you to run to the bathroom more often, but within about five to seven days, your body will settle and bathroom breaks will taper off.

The average adult needs approximately sixty-four ounces or more of water per day. Of course, if it's hotter outside, you exercise, or you are pregnant or lactating, you'll need more.

The easiest way to figure out how much you need is by dividing your body weight by two. For example, if you weigh 150 pounds, divide that by two and get seventy-five.

Filtered water is ideal, but water can also come from tea, broth, and water-rich fruits and vegetables, such as watermelon and strawberries.

You'll know if you are dehydrated by simply feeling thirsty, having a dry mouth, dry lips, nausea, fatigue, light-headedness, darkening urine color, or decreased urination. When you travel, drink a little extra water before and during your flight. The air is much drier during a flight than on the ground. A flight of more than two hours puts you at risk for dehydration.

On hot days, carry your water with you and sip it regularly. As for strenuous exercise, plan on drinking one cup of water for every fifteen minutes of exercise. Consider adding "Rehydration" homeopathic drops by a company called Energetix to your water bottle to maintain your mineral balance. You can find it on Amazon.

To make it even more enjoyable, add a little flavor. You can add lemon slices, peppermint sprigs, or the supplement powder Glyteine from the list of cleansing supplements.

Key Points

- Water is essential to help your body release toxins.
- Take water with you wherever you go to stay hydrated.
- Drink three to four of your thirty-four ounce water bottles daily.

Put it Into Practice

Now that you know why hydration is essential, calculate how much you need each day and challenge yourself to drink the total amount. Add one of the suggested flavorings to make your water taste better. Carry your water with you wherever you go.

Prayer

Lord, thank you for giving me access to clean water and the desire to enjoy it so I feel better overall. I pray that it blesses my body and thoroughly cleanses it from the inside out. Amen.

Affirmation

Write down the following affirmation, take a deep breath, clear any negative thoughts, say it out loud *three* times, and allow it to sink deep into your heart:

> "I carry my water with me and am well hydrated. I enjoy drinking plenty of pure water."

Checkup

You made it almost to the end of the most challenging part. Now it's time to press on and make it stick. Journal about what's been most challenging and why it's so important to keep going.

TYPES OF SUGARS TO AVOID

It is not good to eat too much honey.

—Proverbs 25:27

Reflect

Have your cravings diminished? If so, that's awesome. Next we'll focus on sugar hidden in food. Sugar can be from a natural source of plants (fruits, honey, molasses), and some starchy vegetables (corn, coconut, potatoes, or sugar cane).

But processed sugar is a big concern. This is a list of the most common types of processed sugar.

- Dextrose
- Maltose
- Brown sugar
- Evaporated cane juice
- Malt syrup
- Cane crystals

- Fructose
- Cane sugar
- Fruit juice concentrates
- Coconut sugar
- Glucose
- Raw sugar
- Corn sweetener
- High-fructose corn syrup
- Sucrose
- Corn syrup
- Syrup
- Crystalline fructose
- Invert sugar
- Agave nectar

Although sugars go by many names, whether processed or natural, they all contain four calories per gram and are metabolized similarly in your body. The exceptions to those are alternative, low-calorie, or no-calorie, sweeteners. These sweeteners can be more addictive than natural sugar because of their extremely high level of sweetness compared to raw or granulated sugar.

I suggest you hold off on all processed sugars and limit yourself to only one to two servings of low glycemic sugars (fruit) per the provided meal plan. Use these tips to reduce overall added sugar intake:

1. Enjoy plain yogurt with no added sugar. For added sweetness, stir in fresh or no-sugar-added frozen fruit and a dash of cinnamon.

2. Look for water, tea, coffee, seltzer, and other beverages with no added sugar. Add a slice of orange, lemon, lime, or cucumber for a little extra flavor.

3. When a sweet craving hits, grab one cup of ripe strawberries or a one-ounce square of 85 percent dark chocolate, and add a tablespoon of unsweetened nut butter for a little boost of healthy fat and protein.

4. No matter what you choose, chew slowly and savor it. Chewing activates the sensors in your body to tell it to get prepared for incoming food. It's essential to chew when drinking smoothies and fresh pressed juices to get complete nutrient absorption.

5. See how your taste buds can adjust to sweetness levels. As you focus on consistently reducing your total sugar intake, you will see your sweet cravings lessen and certain foods now taste too sweet.

Key Points

- Avoid processed sugar.
- Limit fruits to one serving per day.

Put it Into Practice

Keep up with your meal plan and enjoy natural food alternatives to manage sweet treat cravings. Eat plain yogurt with cinnamon and fresh fruit, a cup of strawberries, or a one-ounce square of 85 percent dark chocolate.

Prayer

Lord, thank you for the wisdom to know the difference between types of sugars, what to look for and what to avoid in my diet. Help me put you before my tastebuds. Allow my tastebuds to quickly adjust to new flavors that benefit my health. Thank you, Lord, for being on this journey with me. I love that we are doing this together. I love you, Lord. Amen.

Affirmation

Write down the following affirmation, take a deep breath, clear any negative thoughts, say it out loud *three* times, and allow it to sink deep into your heart:

> "I know what to look for on labels when it comes to sugar, and I am eager to taste new things."

Checkup

Are you still on track? What have been the keys to your success so far?

____

____

____

____

WHY YOU NEED CARBS

Then you will know the truth,
and the truth will set you free.

—John 8:32

Reflect

This twenty-one-day cleanse is about eliminating carbohydrate sugar. But it's not a good idea to eliminate carbs completely. Carbs are your primary energy source, especially for brain function.

They can be used for immediate energy or stored in our liver and muscles for a sustained energy source, healthy digestion, and bowel movements.

Three main types of carbohydrates exist: sugar, fiber, and starch. Simple sugars occur naturally in milk (lactose) and fruit (fructose). The most common simple sugars added to foods include raw sugar, brown sugar, corn syrup, high fructose corn syrup, glucose, fructose, and sucrose. Added sugars are often hidden and may catch you by surprise.

Foods with added sugars are bread (even some brown ones), yogurt, cereals, granola, marinara sauce, dried fruit, ketchup, dips, sauces, coffee drinks (flavored and occasionally "plain" flavor), sweetened iced tea, barbeque sauce, salad dressings, and sweetened fruit juice.

Unfortunately, the bacteria in your body loves to feed on sugar. When you fight a cold or bacterial infection and want to feel better, you must eliminate simple sugars to kill off the bug.

Complex carbohydrates also are found in fiber and starches. They are higher in fiber and promote healthy digestion and regular, smooth bowel movements. Some examples include sprouted grain bread, peas, beans, fruit, and vegetables.

Some people think starchy foods are fattening, but gram for gram, they contain fewer than half the calories of fat. Weight gain is more about varying blood sugar levels throughout the day and the toxin buildup in fat cells than calories.

The cleanse meal plan created for this program is low carb and allows you to focus on plant foods and lean meats to support the detoxification process.

Key Points

- During the cleanse and beyond, make sure your carbs are from whole food (i.e., fruit, veggies, natural sourdough, or whole wheat) to keep your gut healthy, maintain energy and strengthen your immune system.
- Feel refreshed and revitalized without sugar.

Put it Into Practice

Reflect and discover the benefit of trading out simple carbohydrates with the complex ones included in the meal plan.

Avoid reaching for sugary snacks for energy. Instead, go for a walk or get in your daily workout. Or you may find you need to recharge or rest, even if it's just for five minutes. Grab a tall glass of water and take ten to fifteen minutes to slowly sip and breathe. Close your eyes and rest.

Prayer

Thank you, Lord, for the truth and for living free from being afraid of eating carbohydrates, but knowing how they can serve my body. Thank you for creating food that my body needs to be its best, and that I can make choices to feel my best and bring you glory, God. Amen.

Affirmation

Write down the following affirmation, take a deep breath, clear any negative thoughts, say it out loud *three* times, and allow it to sink deep into your heart:

> "I am no longer afraid of carbs. I know the truth."

Checkup

Almost halfway there. Take it one day at a time. What has surprised you the most about this experience so far?

____

____

____

____

ALCOHOL

But he said to me, "My grace is sufficient for you, for
my power is made perfect in weakness." Therefore I will
boast all the more gladly about my weaknesses,
so that Christ's power may rest on me.

—2 Corinthians 12:9

Reflect

How do you feel about eliminating alcohol? Some people can take it or leave. For others, it's a challenge to go without.

In the early days of offering my "Sugar Detox" course, many clients were all-in for getting rid of sugar but struggled with giving up alcohol. One woman felt restricted when she realized that over the twenty-one days of the detox, she had already made previous plans to celebrate with friends one night.

She became frustrated. She wanted to have a fun night out and enjoy drinks and dessert with her friends. She was upfront with me and said she wanted to rebel.

That night she drank a cocktail. The next day she admitted her disappointment because she realized she could have done without the alcohol and felt she let herself down. She decided to stick to the plan and give up alcohol for the next twenty-one days.

Another woman was ready to give up sugar but couldn't see herself giving up beer. She opted out of the program. Alcohol, like sugar, elevates dopamine levels that make you feel happier. Other people turn to alcohol to calm nerves and anxiety.

Sugar and alcohol are associated with celebrations, bonding with others, and a way to relax and unwind. Interestingly enough, they also metabolize in our bodies in similar ways.

During this cleanse, you must refrain from alcohol because of its high sugar content and toxic effects on your body. Drinking alcohol regularly—even just one to two times per week—can cause you to crave sugar.

When your liver metabolizes alcohol, it produces a toxin called acetaldehyde, which causes your skin to become dehydrated and age prematurely. This causes more breakouts and wrinkles. Alcohol also causes bloating.

While on your journey, giving up alcohol may be more difficult than expected. The idea of having it taken away can make you want it that much more. We will always want more of the things we can't have. You don't have to be sad and feel sorry for yourself about losing alcohol. Here's a list of fun alternatives:

- Hot or cold tea.
- Sparkling water with lime.
- Cranberry-pomegranate juice with sparkling water.

- Tonic water with fresh fruit or lime, or a fresh sprig of rosemary or thyme.

- Use zero-proof spirits or soda water as a base and add fresh fruit, such as oranges, strawberries, lemon, lime, or pomegranate seeds.

- Unsweetened coffee, black coffee, latte with unsweetened milk or added flavors, or Americano with unsweetened almond milk or espresso.

Key Point

- Choose fun alternatives to alcoholic beverages.

Put it Into Practice

You don't have to mourn the loss of alcohol. Instead, choose fun alternatives, especially when you go out with friends.

Do something for yourself for kicks. Try something new and fun for you to do.

Prayer

Lord, I know that using alcohol to calm my anxiety and distress—or fit in with friends—isn't the wisest path for me. In those times, I need to be reminded to seek you and find rest for my soul. I am thankful for alternatives that honor my body as a temple of the Holy Spirit. Amen.

Affirmation

Write down the following affirmation, take a deep breath, clear any negative thoughts, say it out loud *three* times, and allow it to sink deep into your heart:

> "I can enjoy tasty non-alcoholic drinks and am excited
> to try new things."

Checkup

Have you stayed on course? If not, jump back in from where you left off and keep going. Journal your thoughts.

____

____

____

____

ARTIFICIAL AND NATURAL LOW-CALORIE SWEETENERS

Do not conform to the pattern of this world,
but be transformed by the renewing of your mind.
Then you will be able to test and approve what God's
will is—his good, pleasing, and perfect will.

—Romans 12:2

Reflect

Do you feel better? Have your cravings gone away?

Around days seven to ten, your cravings should have diminished significantly. Let's discuss low-calorie sweeteners and why to avoid them.

Many of my clients asked me if they could have artificial or natural low-calorie sweeteners during their cleanse. When you detox sugar, it's easy to want artificial sweeteners as an alternative. You want to enjoy something sweet without the calories—all the pleasure without the guilt. As usual, anything too good to be true has consequences. This is the case with artificial sweeteners.

Artificial sweeteners are manufactured sugar substitutes. They often are much sweeter than natural sugar and lead to more frequent cravings.

A friend became addicted to Diet Pepsi. Every day after work she stopped at the vending machine in her apartment building. She felt an uncontrollable urge and had no idea why. She was healthy, fit, and thought she was doing the right thing by getting a diet soda to avoid extra sugar and calories. Unfortunately she became hooked on the intense sweetness.

Some studies with laboratory animals have found a link between artificial sweeteners–such as saccharin and aspartame–and cancer. According to the National Cancer Institute and the Cancer Council, recent studies suggest that although animal studies caused bladder cancer and increased the risk of cancer in the offspring of pregnant rats, they couldn't prove it had the same effect on people.[5]

However, in my opinion, if there is any cancer risk, I would avoid saccharin and aspartame.

One small packet of Splenda can kill two-thirds of your healthy gut bacteria. Nutrasweet is a neurotoxin, which means it's toxic to your brain.

---

[5] National Cancer Institute, "Artificial Sweeteners and Cancer," National Cancer Institute, August 10, 2016, https://www.cancer.gov/about-cancer/causes-prevention/risk/diet/artificial-sweeteners-fact-sheet#is-there-an-association-between-artificial-sweeteners-and-cancer

Artificial sweeteners don't contain calories because they are indigestible. Researchers previously assumed that, because they are indigestible, they have no effect on gut health. Recent research, however, shows that gut bacteria is compromised.[6] In mice, researchers have found a link between sucralose and its adverse effects on gut bacteria. Since gut bacteria is responsible for healthy digestion and immune function, it must be protected.

Another issue is that artificial sweeteners tend to produce gas, bloating, cramping, and diarrhea in some people, especially anyone suffering from irritable bowel syndrome or other digestive sensitivities.

The following list will help you identify the most common artificial (chemical) sweeteners. You should avoid all of them.

- Aspartame (Nutrasweet)
- Sucralose (Splenda)
- Acesulfame K (Sunett)
- Saccharin (Sweet Twin, Sweet 'N Low)

Several low-calorie plant-based sweeteners—Stevia, Erythritol, and Xylitol—seem healthier, but we also will exclude them during our cleanse. These alternative sweeteners are low in calories, low in fructose (fruit sugar), and taste very sweet. Unfortunately, they lead to an increased desire for sugar.

____

[6] Francisco Javier Ruiz-Ojeda, Julio Plaza-Díaz, Maria Jose Sáez-Lara, and Angel Gil, "Effects of Sweeteners on the Gut Microbiota: A Review of Experimental Studies and Clinical Trials, January 10, 2019, https://www.ncbi.nlm.nih.gov/pmc/articles/PMC6363527/

Stevia is sweet and leaves you with a bitter aftertaste that prevents many from using it. Erythritol is a sugar alcohol found naturally in certain fruits. But it can cause digestive issues, including gas and diarrhea, if you consume too much at one time, especially if it's combined with other types of sugar such as fructose. Xylitol is also very sweet and, like other sugar alcohols, can cause high doses of digestive side effects, including abdominal gas and diarrhea.

Instead, use a touch of honey or cinnamon as you wean off sugar.

Key Points

- Avoid artificial sweeteners.
- For this cleanse, refrain from artificial and plant-based, low-calorie sweeteners so you can completely reset your palate.
- Use alternatives–a teaspoon of honey or cinnamon–to curb cravings.

Put it Into Practice

If you need a little sweetness, you can choose one teaspoon of honey or cinnamon in hot drinks or on apples to reduce sugar cravings.

Prayer

Thank you, Lord, for the natural sweetness in the plants you gave us here on earth. I choose to enjoy the natural sweetness you created for us. Amen.

Affirmation

Write down the following affirmation, take a deep breath, clear any negative thoughts, say it out loud *three* times, and allow it to sink deep into your heart:

"I choose to live without chemically-created artificial sweeteners as an investment in my health."

Checkup

You have gone more than ten days without sugar and with plenty of healthy whole food. You should feel clean, refreshed, revitalized, and energized. How are you feeling?

NUTRITION BASICS

Everything that lives and moves about will be food for
you. Just as I gave you the green plants,
I now give you everything.

—Genesis 9:3

Reflect

Having a preset meal plan and being guided on precisely what to eat is helpful, especially if you have a busy lifestyle that leaves you without extra time to think. Although you have a plan in place, you may need help for when the detox is over.

I remember praying, reflecting, and asking God how we should eat. I believe he showed me that we should eat mostly plants, along with a smaller portion of animal products. Fish, eggs, lamb, and some poultry options in smaller amounts are ideal.

I received confirmation of these principles by noticing how good my clients felt by eating this way. They were naturally cleansing toxins from their bodies and hitting the "reset" button on their health. I was amazed at how many broke free from allergy-related congestion, postnasal drip, abdominal bloating, joint pain, skin rashes, acne, excess body fat, low energy, headaches, and poor sleep.

My clients could breathe easier, think more clearly, and move easily. Many lost the stubborn extra layer of fat. As a result, I was inspired to create the 21-Day Sugar Detox program, which allowed many to heal their bodies from the inside-out using a paleo-style meal plan that is composed of 30 percent whole food carbohydrate, 30 percent protein, and 40 percent healthy plant-based fats.

I know plenty of diet programs, such as keto and juice fast cleanses, which heavily limit protein or carbohydrates. Unfortunately, I've seen many people struggle to maintain a keto diet because it lacks the carbohydrates we need. Fasting eliminates protein vital to our well-being.

Restricting carbs eventually leads to overindulgence. Your brain, cardiovascular system, kidneys, and muscular system run on carbohydrates for energy. Your hormone and nervous systems run on healthy fats. Your body's structure and immune system depend on protein as its foundation.

Your body also needs micronutrients such as vitamins and minerals from fruits, whole grains, and vegetables for immune system health, neuromuscular function, brain health, bone health, and proper growth and development.

A diet rich in various colorful plant foods will naturally provide you with all the necessary micronutrients (vitamins and minerals) and detoxing you desire.

Put it Into Practice

Enjoy the ease of following the meal plan knowing that you are getting the variety of foods you need for health and cleansing.

Prayer

Thank you, Lord, for the food in nature. I want more of the foods that fulfill all of my physical needs and give you glory. Amen.

Affirmation

Write down the following affirmation, take a deep breath, clear any negative thoughts, say it out loud *three* times, and allow it to sink deep into your heart:

> "I am thankful to eat a balanced diet filled with colorful plant foods."

Checkup

It should not surprise you that you have read this far into the book. This program was made for you. Now is your time. Make the most of it. Journal your thoughts for today.

FIBER AND DETOXING

Then God said, "I give you every seed-bearing plant
on the face of the whole earth and every tree with fruit
with seed. They will be yours for food."

—Genesis 1:29

Reflect

Have you ever felt you ate healthy but didn't understand why you felt bloated and full of intermittent gas pain, especially after eating a big salad, raw veggies, nuts, or beans?

As you probably have already figured out, this program's meal plan contains plenty of fiber. You also may have noticed a little extra bloating or gassiness within the first week. If you ate primarily plant foods before you began our journey together, you might not have felt much of a change.

These plant foods are our primary source of fiber. Along with plenty of water, fiber aids in the healthy flow of digestion and elimination. Our gut contains billions of bacteria that must be fed healthy fiber from green leafy veggies and various plants daily.

A common condition known as "leaky gut" can set in without adequate fiber. A "leaky gut" causes inflammation and produces several physical symptoms: chronic constipation, skin rashes or acne, eczema, food allergies, a depleted immune system, bloating, joint and abdominal pain, headache, fatigue, difficulty concentrating, and chronic diarrhea.

In an article from UCLA Health by Elizabeth Ko, MD, and Eve Glazier, MD, they state, "The best protection is a healthful diet high in natural fiber and low in added sugars and processed foods. It's also important to go easy on the alcohol and to get daily exercise."[7]

Fiber helps you to feel full after meals and with weight loss. Eating three to five daily servings of fruits and veggies is ideal.

This might sound expensive, but it's not. You don't have to spend a ton of money on organic produce. Only a select few need to be organic.

The produce that must be organic is affectionately known as the "Dirty Dozen." These should be "certified organic" or bought from a certified organic farm stand at your local farmers market.

The complete list of the foods in the "Dirty Dozen" Category as identified by the Environmental Working Group (EWG):

1. Strawberries

2. Spinach

3. Kale, collard, and mustard greens

---

[7] Elizabeth Ko, MD, and Eve Glazier, MD, "Ask the Doctors – Just why is fiber good for you?," UCLA Health Ask the Doctors, June 29,2018, https://connect.uclahealth.org/2018/06/29/ask-the-doctors-just-why-is-fiber-good-for-you/

4. Nectarines
5. Apples
6. Grapes
7. Bell and hot peppers
8. Cherries
9. Peaches
10. Pears
11. Celery
12. Tomatoes

Eating more plant foods in place of sugary treats will give you the fiber, vitamins, and minerals you need to reduce cravings. Opting for low-sugar fruits such as berries, peaches, lemons and limes, honeydew melon, oranges, grapefruit, and avocado is your best bet for keeping blood sugar levels in check and reducing the risk for refined sugar cravings.

When upping fiber in your diet, drink plenty of fluids. When fiber travels through your digestive tract, it's like a new sponge. It needs water to plump up and pass through smoothly. Eating more fiber than usual without enough fluid can lead to nausea or constipation.

Key Point

- Fiber keeps your gut healthy, makes you feel full, and helps remove toxins from your body.

Put it Into Practice

Since the meal plan is high in fiber, drink plenty of water (half of your body weight in ounces) to help it move through your digestive tract more efficiently.

Prayer

Lord, thank you for the plants of the earth for giving me a healthy body. I look forward to experiencing all the health benefits of the foods you created for me to eat as a perfect match for my body. Amen.

Affirmation

Write down the following affirmation, take a deep breath, clear any negative thoughts, say it out loud *three* times, and allow it to sink deep into your heart:

> "Fiber is integral to my digestive and overall health.
> I am excited to see how it helps to keep me full and
> cleansed from the inside out."

Checkup

Name something you have overcome that has made you feel proud of yourself.

EXERCISE

Do not be wise in your own eyes; fear the Lord and shun evil. This will bring health to your body and nourishment to your bones.

—Proverbs 3:7-8

Reflect

Do you love or loathe exercise? Chances are, if the only reason you exercise is to conform to a certain body image, you are on an emotional roller coaster. The right reason to exercise is to care for the body God gave you and to feel better.

Media messages can be confusing. In one commercial, you see a beautifully thin and fit woman who is successful and leads a vibrant life. You see mannequins of all shapes and sizes where we buy clothes. Larger ones wear T-shirts touting "embrace your curves" or "love your body." Tall, thin ones that look cute in every outfit.

Where are examples of someone in-between? Why do we have to fall into one category or the other?

Whatever your shape, you are perfectly designed and handcrafted with God's love. If someone created a beautiful work of art for you, wouldn't you want to take care of it? Doing so would signify gratitude and love for the creator.

Wellness and beauty aren't about your body size or shape but rather how you treat your body. Like anything else, the better you treat your body, the better it will treat you. You will have a natural glow, more energy, look younger, and reflect the Lord.

Conversely, if you are sedentary, eat mainly processed foods, and feel constantly frustrated, your life will reflect that. Ultimately, you have to choose.

As a young adult in college, I lived with constant fear and anxiety about what I ate, how I looked, and what others thought of me. I am a natural leader and wanted to ensure I looked my best so others would look up to me for being consistent with exercise and eating healthy.

No matter how much I worked out and limited the foods in my diet, it was never enough. I ignored my body and stayed numb from emotions. I worked hard with weights, cardio, and counting calories. The Lord continued to love me anyway. He stuck by me when I ignored him and wanted to be in complete control. I was "chasing the wind," as described in Ecclesiastes. I chased perfection but could never capture it long enough to feel complete.

With professional counseling, prayer, and healing, the Lord brought me out of misery and into freedom. I had to give up exercise and food as an idol to break free. I had to repent and ask for forgiveness and healing.

Exercising too much isn't a problem for most. Ultimately, it's about self-care and bringing glory to God. You must ask yourself, "Is this only for me, or is this for God too? Can I make it for God too?" Why not begin to view exercise as a heartfelt act of worship and gratitude?

Exercise is known for calming the mind and relieving stress. It naturally boosts endorphins, energy, and brain chemicals like dopamine. Instead of reaching for sugar, go for a walk.

There are a million reasons why exercise is essential. It has an anti-aging effect, and encourages fat loss and lean muscle gain. It helps your clothes fit better, so you feel more confident. Exercise helps you stand taller, breathe easier, and strengthen bones and your immune system. It promotes excellent sleep, improved intimacy with your spouse, and body confidence in the bedroom. You'll find that you are happier, have a better attitude, and feel beautiful.

Being fit and healthy will allow you to be readily available for what God calls you to do. You will have the energy and vitality he needs you to have to do it. In addition, you will be a vibrant and beautiful reflection of his kingdom.

Cling to the Lord for help to stay consistent. Knowing you are doing it as an act of worship and bringing God glory is a good place to start. Take it one workout at a time, and you will realize how good you feel every time you complete a workout.

You need about four to six weeks of consistent, well-planned workouts to see significant results. But when you see those results, it's great motivation to keep going.

Even before you workout , set a long-term vision for yourself. How do you want to look and feel? Journaling your description and draw a picture of what it would look like for you. Claim it daily.

After you have your long-term vision, set up short-term goals to achieve your ultimate dream. Grab a calendar and set small weekly goals. Mark your calendar by crossing off each workout when you complete it.

Focus on doing your best with each workout. Before you know it, you will have established a healthy routine. You'll feel good about yourself, and notice the physical changes that will make you want to return for more.

I recommend at least three days of strength training with weights or body weight to start. Include two days of heart-pumping cardio, one day of stretching, and one day off. Start somewhere, even if it's just going outside your door and taking a walk.

The hardest part is getting started, so be sure to plan the night before. Some people even go to bed in their workout clothes as a built-in reminder to exercise as soon as they wake up. Typically, the best time to work out is first thing in the morning, although you may find your best time is after work.

Check out my sample workout calendar here: www.wellwithinutrition.com/free-21-day-fitness-plan

You can also join one of my online "21-Day Fitness and Nutrition Challenge Groups" for fun, accountability, community, daily education, inspiration, and structure: www.wellwithinutrition.com/21-fitness-nutrition-challenge

Key Points

- Take good care of your body. It is the temple of the Holy Spirit.
- Move regularly.
- Use exercise to reduce cravings and manage stress.
- Exercise keeps you young, is a form of worship, and helps remove toxins.

Put it Into Practice

Make a workout plan. Go for a twenty- to thirty-minute walk three times a week, do strength workouts three times per week, and stretch once a week. Keep it simple and use the workout calendar featured on my website.

Prayer

Lord, sustaining my workouts even when I have the best intentions can be challenging. But you can help me to see the benefits of exercise on my mental health, so I can feel and look better. Help me keep going so I can better reflect you. Amen.

Affirmation

Write down the following affirmation, take a deep breath, clear any negative thoughts, say it out loud *three* times, and allow it to sink deep into your heart:

> "I will exercise regularly as unto the Lord, freeing my
> mind, strengthening my body, and invigorating my soul
> for your glory."

Checkup

It's time to get moving. It's up to you. Make the decision today to move. Jot down your workout plan below.

HORMONES AND SUGAR

So do not fear, for I am with you; do not be dismayed,
for I am your God. I will strengthen and help you; I will
uphold you with my righteous right hand.

—Isaiah 41:10

Reflect

Hormonal imbalances and changes can make removing sugar from your diet difficult. Premenstrual Syndrome (PMS) each month is a thing for me and probably for you. Symptoms are individual and vary a bit from month to month, especially as you get older and after having kids. During this time, cravings are usually specific, such as a strong desire for chocolate, baked goods, ice cream, and carbohydrate and fat-laden foods.

Fluctuations in cortisol and estrogen levels are the main culprit for these symptoms. Cortisol and estrogen work interchangeably. When cortisol is high, estrogen is low, and when estrogen is high, cortisol is low. Weeks before your period, estrogen increases, and you experience premenstrual symptoms. When estrogen decreases, cortisol, also known as the stress hormone, goes up. Your body is put into a state of high stress, which leads to an increased appetite and cravings for fat and carbs.

Serotonin, a brain chemical which makes you feel good, can also cause sugar cravings. When serotonin levels dip, it can affect food cravings during PMS.

When your cortisol is high and serotonin levels are low, you become more likely to crave simple and sugary carbohydrates, such as chocolate.

On the other hand, if your cortisol levels are high and serotonin is within normal levels, you will likely crave foods high in fat and carbs, such as ice cream and brownies. Healthy sources of fats such as Omega-3 work to rebuild cells and keep hormone levels stable.

Magnesium is another mineral you can quickly become deficient in and not even realize it. Low magnesium levels can significantly impact PMS symptoms, such as headaches, cramping, and cravings. To alleviate hormone-related migraines, soak in a magnesium bath with Epsom salts, the salt form of magnesium. A bath is a natural way to allow the salt to enter your body through your skin as you soothe your body and soul.

If baths aren't your thing, you can enjoy a warm magnesium drink. I like to use the powder form of Natural Calm Magnesium from Natural Vitality. The powder can be found on Amazon or at your local health food or supplement store. Magnesium also is excellent for alleviating menstrual cramps and sugar cravings. Since magnesium relaxes nerves and muscles, it will help relax uterine muscles and relieve cramping.

As for chocolate cravings, research has shown this is an indication your body is crying out for magnesium. Make sure you get enough magnesium to help combat chocolate cravings. Dark chocolate (85 percent or higher cocoa content) is exceptionally high in magnesium and antioxidants and can make a great PMS snack.

Let's not forget irritability, anger, and sadness during your period. Magnesium is known to calm nerves. It can even boost your mood since it plays a role in the production of serotonin.

Magnesium-rich foods—almonds, dark chocolate, popcorn, and pumpkin seeds—are perfect snacks during your premenstrual time.

You may wonder if giving in to your PMS cravings is okay. As you've learned, cravings are your body's way of telling you that it needs to get back into a balanced hormonal state. However, food cravings are only a temporary fix that could lead to a blood sugar crash. The best way to combat cravings is to give your body what it truly needs— more magnesium, healthy fats, rest, physical activity, and balanced meals.

Key Points

- Hormones affect cravings.
- Chocolate cravings can be caused by a magnesium deficiency.

Put it Into Practice

Since hormone fluctuations can cause irregular moods and sugar cravings, have magnesium on hand for a bath or a warm drink.

Prayer

Lord, help me when tempted to give in to my cravings. I know I have a choice, and I can choose to walk away or find a non-sugar whole food alternative to fulfill my nutritional needs. Amen.

Affirmation

Write down the following affirmation, take a deep breath, clear any negative thoughts, say it out loud *three* times, and allow it to sink deep into your heart:

> "I will become more mindful of my cravings when they coincide with my cycle."

Checkup

Hormones can be tricky. What have you learned that can help you understand yours better?

____

____

____

____

HOW TO COMBAT EMOTIONAL EATING

Come to me, all you who are weary and burdened, and I will give you rest. Take my yoke upon you and learn from me, for I am gentle and humble in heart, and you will find rest for your souls. For my yoke is easy and my burden is light.

—Matthew 11:28-30

Reflect

Emotional eating is eating to soothe uncomfortable feelings and emotions. Food is meant to satisfy physical hunger, not fill emotional needs. Emotional eating is triggered when something upsets you. The picture of a donut or brownie may pass through your mind, and you crave it. You cannot let go of the feeling until you eat one.

Are you an Emotional Eater?

- Do you eat more when you're stressed?
- Do you eat when you're not hungry?

- Do you reward yourself with food?
- Do you regularly eat until you've stuffed yourself?
- Does food make you feel safe? Do you feel like food is a friend?
- Do you feel powerless or out of control around food?[8]

We must remember the spiritual aspect of emotional eating. Ask the Holy Spirit to reveal the spiritual battle taking place. Ask someone who has been delivered from emotional eating to pray over you so you, too, can be free.

Being physically hungry and looking for a stress reliever is a deadly combo. For example, you are at home, the house is quiet, the kids are in bed, and you are relaxing and watching your favorite show. The thought of cookies, ice cream, or a glass of wine appears in your mind. You think a treat might be the perfect ending to the day. You pause your show, grab the treat, cuddle up with a blanket on the couch, and resume your show. You eat and watch but barely notice the taste. You fall asleep on the sofa, but are later awakened by a loud commercial. You turn off the TV and climb into bed. The following day you wake up with a sugar hangover. The guilt kicks in, and you swear off all sugar.

Overeating sugar usually happens at night. Emotional cravings typically occur because you want connection, a break, or a moment of bliss. Ask God to show you healthier ways to meet your legitimate emotional needs. Make a list of things you find emotionally satisfying and put them on your calendar.

---

[8] Melinda Smith, M.A., Lawrence Robinson, Jeanne Segal Ph.D., and Robert Segal, M.A. "Emotional Eating and How to Stop It," Health Guide: Your trusted nonprofit guide to mental health & wellness, August 30, 2022

Other times, cravings can come after meals when you simply want to change the taste on your palate. This is called "food monotony." The main goal in alleviating food monotony is merely changing the taste in your mouth after eating a savory meal. To do that, chew on sugar-free mint gum, brush your teeth, have some tea or coffee, grab some 85 percent dark chocolate or hot lemon water, or rinse with mouthwash or water.

Studies show food is often related to our strongest memories. Sugary treats especially carry fond memories of connecting with family during a celebration, parties, vacations, and fun times. We reach for a sugary treat when we want to rekindle that "fuzzy" feeling.

Emotional hunger and physical hunger are different.

Emotional eating is spontaneous, specific, and constant until you satisfy the urge. it's mainly felt in your head, mouth, or the surface of your thoughts. It's hard to completely satisfy and often leads to feeling uncomfortably full.

Physical hunger starts gradually. You feel it physically within your stomach, a growling pain that comes in waves. You are open to several options, even less palatable foods, and it's easy to satisfy with an average amount of food.

When you feel physically hungry, your body tells you it needs fuel. Emotional hunger can come on quickly, and one cannot be satisfied with food. You leave the experience with physical pain, feelings of disgust and shame, and emotions that drove you to eat in the first place.[9]

---

[9] Eric Chowles, "6 Differences Between Emotional and Physical Hunger," Sleek Geek Health Revolution, 2022, https://www.sleekgeek.co.za/2017/06/hunger/

You can often identify emotions based on the foods you choose to eat. For example:

Crunchy Salty Foods: Craving emotional release, usually when experiencing anger/boredom, frustration, or anxiety.

Sweet Creamy Foods: Craving comfort, wanting a hug or affirmation, feeling sad, lonely, or scared.

Sugar and dopamine are heavily linked. When an individual eats sugar, the brain produces enormous surges of dopamine. This is similar to how the brain reacts to ingesting heroin and cocaine.

Researchers think this might be because our bodies have adapted to seek foods high in calories.

For most of human history, eating many calories was essential to survive. With modern food technology and the widespread availability of high-calorie foods, at least in Western nations, this is no longer necessary for survival.

The first step to conquering emotional eating is to identify your common triggers. What was happening in your life, and what were the emotions you were experiencing? The most common trigger feelings are feeling too hungry, angry, lonely, stressed/overwhelmed, and very tired.

When you identify your trigger emotions, you will see that food cannot satisfy the need. You need a distraction and a sense of connection to your feelings, your body, God, or someone else around you to whom you can reach out to. Make a firm decision that you will not eat unless you are physically hungry and emotionally grounded.

The next time you find yourself craving sweets and experiencing emotional eating, tell yourself to *stop*. Step away from food for thirty minutes and take five deep breaths. Then ask yourself, "What am I feeling, and what do I need right now?"

Ask the Lord for help and to shower you with his love and peace and to speak truth to you. Connect with him and step into peace.

In those thirty minutes, get out of your head by reaching out to a friend, journaling, going for a walk, organizing your purse, drawer, or closet, engaging in meditative breathing, or watching a video that makes you laugh.

Tell yourself you can have the sweet treat when the cleanse is complete, but for now, you will be okay and on your way.

Before each day, commit that if a sugar craving arises, you have a plan in place on how to handle it. Resolve to not give in while you check in with your hunger and emotions.

Key Points

- Learn to combat emotional eating.
- Have a plan in place for dealing with emotional eating.

Put it Into Practice

Begin to distinguish between emotional eating and physical hunger. You will need first to figure out your emotional triggers. When you have that knowledge, you will be on your way to combating it.

Prayer

Lord, I know I do not need to live as a slave to anything because you have set me free. I can turn to you for the strength I need. You can fill the emptiness in my heart when I feel tempted by food. Amen.

Affirmation

Write down the following affirmation, take a deep breath, clear any negative thoughts, say it out loud *three* times, and allow it to sink deep into your heart:

> "Food, especially sugar, is not my master, and I choose
> to serve the Lord."

Checkup

Emotional eating is a complex and serious topic. What emotions do you need to deal with and overcome?

EAT REGULARLY TO LIMIT SUGAR CRAVINGS

Worship the Lord your God, and his blessing will be on your food and water. I will take away sickness from you.

—Exodus 23:25

Reflect

Have you ever found yourself so focused on a task that you forgot to eat? You found yourself with low blood sugar, super hungry, and craving something sweet or "carby." You grabbed a cookie or two or three that left you with a sugar headache, nausea, and guilt because of what you just ate.

You'll need to be prepared to escape the "forgetting to eat" trigger. Your body's natural survival response to low blood sugar is an intense desire for sugar.

Eating well-balanced meals on the meal plan is essential to avoid blood sugar dips and sugar cravings. A good meal includes protein, healthy fat (avocado, olive oil, nuts), veggies, and carbohydrates (starch or fruit).

Planning is key to your success.

The night before, as part of your bedtime routine, plan out your next day, including your exercise and meals. Getting up and starting your day without a plan can lead to stress. If you're not careful, you can find yourself running and chasing the clock.

Take control of your day instead of being controlled by it. We can't predict everything that will happen in a day, but we can make a plan. God's plans may differ from ours, but we plan so we are prepared for anything that may happen..

I recommend to my clients that they carry a "gas can" (extra fuel) of dry snacks—in a purse or glove box—and a full water bottle at all times. Having backup snacks and water is perfect in case of food emergencies.

To start your day off on the right foot, include "you time" in your morning routine. Wake up with enough time to spend in prayer and meditation and soak in the presence of the Lord. When I wake up knowing the day will be hectic, I make myself stop and pray, abide in the Lord's presence, give him all my concerns and worries, and turn the day over to him.

Planning the night before will give you the tools you need to enjoy more health and less stress.

Key Points

- Make sure to include protein and healthy fats to maintain stable blood sugar and keep cravings at bay.
- Take food (fruit or nuts) with you in your backup "gas can."

Plan the night before: what you will eat and the day's workout.

Put it Into Practice

Schedule your tomorrow before you go to bed, including what and when:

- Prayer/meditation/alone with God time
- Workout (what body parts, when, and for how long)
- Supplements
- Breakfast
- Lunch
- Dinner
- Snacks

Prayer

Lord, help me to remember to take the blessing of "food and water" that you have for me and utilize them for my health. It's not always easy to be clear on what I want to eat. But Lord, help me to plan nutritious meals and gain wisdom to fuel my body the best I can. With you, all things are possible, and I look forward to spending intimate time with you before I start my day. Open my eyes to all of the blessings you set before me. Amen

Affirmation

Write down the following affirmation, take a deep breath, clear any negative thoughts, say it out loud *three* times, and allow it to sink deep into your heart:

> "I am 'that' woman who plans to ensure my nutritional success for the next day."

Checkup

Keep going. What changes have you seen? What have others noticed about you?

MINDFUL AND INTUITIVE EATING

And we know that in all things God works for the good
of those who love him, who have been called according
to his purpose.

—Romans 8:28

Reflect

During the past eighteen days of cleansing, you have probably learned much about yourself and your relationship with food. You may have discovered fears and trust issues. You also may have found that you crave healthy whole foods and are more aware of how food makes your body and mind feel.

The concept of mindful and intuitive eating was introduced to me more than twenty years ago. It was a new concept back then but has become a mainstream movement for those who want to break free from dieting. We live in a society of food and body weight extremes. Mindful and intuitive eating helps you to get back into the in-between.

Mindful eating is being mentally and physically present while you eat to experience the taste, texture, temperature, aroma, and colors of your food. Intuitive eating is eating in tune with your body and choosing foods that make you feel your best. Choosing the right foods for your body brings enjoyment, pleasure, a healthy weight, and good health.

Diets provide:

- Rigid structure.
- Putting your total faith in the food combinations.
- Meal frequencies.
- Calorie allotment.

At the same time, mindful and intuitive eating is based on how you feel as a result of the food you eat. For example, feeling tired and sluggish after eating a carby meal instead of feeling light and energized after eating a well-balanced meal with protein, healthy fats, and veggies.

Mindful and intuitive eating takes practice. Nutrition education is necessary to ensure you get the correct balance of healthy foods. It takes trial and error to determine which foods are the best for you. Take a look at the nutrition basics lesson again if you need a little refresher before diving into mindful and intuitive eating.

Dietitian Adda Bjarnadottir, MS, RDN, listed the following tips for mindful eating:

- Eating slowly and without distraction.
- Listening to physical hunger cues and eating until you're full.
- Distinguishing between true hunger and non-hunger triggers for eating.

- Engaging your senses by noticing colors, smells, sounds, textures, and flavors.

- Learning to cope with guilt and anxiety about food.

- Eating to maintain overall health and well-being.

- Noticing the effects food has on your feelings and figure.

- Appreciating your food.[10]

Intuitive eating is a researched-based health approach created in 1995 by two dietitians–Elyse Resch and Evelyn Tribole. Intuitive eating is not a diet because no foods are off-limits, and it is about a return to how you were naturally born to eat. However, our signals could be a lot better. Your appetite may be bigger than it needs to be to stay trim and fit. Our appetites tend to be as big as the amount we eat.

Suppose you remain overweight when eating based on hunger and fullness. You should reduce your overall calorie intake to reset your signals and adapt to slightly fewer calories to maintain a healthy weight.

Ways to practice intuitive eating.

- Stay away from extreme diet fads.

- Listen to your body and honor your hunger.

- Make peace with all foods knowing what works well for you and what doesn't.

---

[10] Adda Bjarnadottir, MS, RDN (Ice), "Mindful Eating 101 — A Beginner's Guide," Healthline Nutrition, June 19, 2019, https://www.healthline.com/nutrition/mindful-eating-guide

- Own your own needs, be confident, and know that what you need now may differ from what used to work or whatever everyone else is doing to lose weight.

- Enjoy discovering how foods satisfy your needs.

- Honor your fullness and enjoy food when you are hungry again.

- Cope with emotions kindly, and know you are growing by allowing yourself to experience them.

- Respect the body God created for you by eating whole foods and exercising regularly.

- Honor your health, and give the Lord glory, honor, and praise.

Mindful and intuitive eating isn't easy, but practice leads to freedom. It allows you to live out your best mental, physical and spiritual health. I encourage you to get back to basics and honor your body's needs with foods that make you feel your best.

Visit my website to learn more about intuitive eating: www.wellwithinutrition.com

Key Points

- Listen to your body's cues for what foods make you feel your best.

- Be intentional about eating and regular exercise.

Put it Into Practice

Learn how to listen to and trust your body when choosing the foods that feel best for you. Make a list of those foods and the ones that don't make you feel great.

Prayer

Lord, I am honored and blessed to have the opportunity to break free into healthy eating and exercise without any strings attached. Give me the wisdom to discern what foods are best for me. If I notice that I am gaining extra weight, open my eyes so I can adjust my nutrition and the number of calories I consume daily. I need your love and support to surround my emotional needs. Thank you for growing me into the person you want me to be. I love you, Lord, and look forward to the transformation that is about to take place. Amen.

Affirmation

Write down the following affirmation, take a deep breath, clear any negative thoughts, say it out loud *three* times, and allow it to sink deep into your heart:

> "I will become mindful of what my body needs."

Checkup

You only have three days to go. How can you incorporate mindful eating today?

PLENTY OF SLEEP

The LORD is my shepherd. I lack nothing. He makes
me lie down in green pastures, he leads me beside quiet
waters, and he refreshes my soul.

—Psalm 23:1-3

Reflect

Rest is sweet, but true refreshment comes when your soul is rested. A refreshed soul brings energy, a zest for life, clear-flowing and creative thoughts, easy breathing, confidence, a sense of peace and tranquility, and a feeling as if you can move mountains.

I've heard it said women are the household's thermostat. If we are tired, overwhelmed, and irritated, so is the rest of the home. By contrast, if we are at peace, rested, confident, secure, and refreshed, everyone else is too. Even without a word spoken, the emotional energy you carry is felt by everyone else, especially those intimately connected with you—your spouse and children.

When feeling stressed, overwhelmed, and exhausted, your body's natural response is to get more energy, usually from rest or food.

If you decide not to rest, you will seek out carbs, caffeine, or both, to keep your brain power and body energy going. The more concentrated the carbs—such as soda, juices, candy, sweetened coffee drinks, and pastries—the more easily they digest, bringing quick energy to your brain, and helping you to stay awake and alert.

Before heading to your stomach, carbohydrates are digested and absorbed through the tissues of your mouth with the help of an enzyme in your saliva called amylase. Unlike protein and fats that are digested and absorbed in your stomach and intestine, carbohydrates produce a calming effect by releasing serotonin into your brain.

In an article published in 2022, Nadia Haris states:

> Eating carbohydrate-rich foods raises the levels of the neurotransmitter serotonin in your brain. This chemical messenger is responsible for feelings of calmness and wellness; low serotonin levels have been linked to depression, anxiety, and insomnia. Hence, eating carbs can be a "feel-good" mechanism regardless of whether you are hungry. By contrast, eating protein-rich foods reduces serotonin levels and increases dopamine and norepinephrine in the brain... Dopamine and norepinephrine enhance alertness, focus, and mental concentration.[11]

It's no wonder we crave sugar when we feel tired or sad. A quick sugar fix gives us a little brain energy boost and makes us feel happy. The energy boost lasts only thirty minutes to one hour before blood sugar and energy crash and a craving returns.

---

[11] Nadia Haris, "How Food Affects Neurotransmitters," SFGATE, 2022, https://healthyeating.sfgate.com/what-ate-lose-weight-noom-13771700.html

My lowest energy moments were in college, grad school, and when the kids were babies. The long days, short nights, and demanding workload took a toll on my body and soul. I still needed to learn how to calm down and reset. The anxiety I struggled with kept me stuck. I was all or nothing. I craved carbs for quick energy and to stay awake.

The endless cycle of lack of sleep, exhaustion, headaches, erratic blood sugar, and carb cravings finally caught up to me. I consulted a psychotherapist and learned how to harness my perfectionist ways, listen to my body, practice daily meditation, and calm my mind without sugary food when I was wound up.

Ultimately I committed to giving my fears to the Lord and asked him to speak his truth. The more I experienced peace, the more I wanted peace. My daily decision to lie down in green pastures by the still water was where I gained freedom from anxiety and began refreshing my soul. As a part of learning to calm myself, I learned how to have a healthy and refreshing sleep.

You need about seven to nine hours of sleep per night. This allows your body to heal, repair, and rejuvenate. You likely will wake up to a restored body and refreshed soul.

To get a restful night's sleep, follow a nightly bedtime routine.

1. Set a time to start your routine, be in bed, and be asleep by 10:00 p.m.

2. Turn off the TV and move portable electronics out of the bedroom. Turn off all screens (including phone and laptop) at least one hour before bed.

3. Drink a warm cup of hot lemon water or herbal tea.

4. Take a shower or bath, put on soft, comfortable pajamas.

5. Brush your teeth (wait at least one hour after drinking lemon water).

6. Read a book or your Bible, spend time in prayer and meditation, and ask God to give you restful sleep to refresh your soul.

7. Ensure the temperature is just right for restful sleep. Lower your thermostat, if need be, and add blankets to keep you warm and cozy, not hot and sweaty.

8. Have a cup or bottle of water on your nightstand.

9. Make sure your room is dark with shades down if you intend to wake up after the sun rises.

When this practice becomes routine, you will see how refreshed you feel. Teach your kids to do the same and hope they continue the routine throughout their life.

Key Point

- Fatigue can cause you to crave sugar. But with a nightly sleep routine, you will feel refreshed, alert, at peace, and ready to conquer your day.

Put it Into Practice

Starting tonight, focus on getting quality sleep. Follow the bedtime routine steps and the wellness routine tips for quality sleep to reduce the risk of sugar cravings and improve your energy.

Prayer

Lord, I am committed to giving myself the sleep I need and deserve. I want to lie in green pastures, be led beside quiet waters, and refresh my soul. Give me the sweet, sweet sleep you have for me so I can be the person you want me to be. Amen.

Affirmation

Write down the following affirmation, take a deep breath, clear any negative thoughts, say it out loud *three* times, and allow it to sink deep into your heart:

> "Every time I close my eyes, I get sweet sleep."

Checkup

Focus tonight on getting some sweet sleep. A great way to sleep well is to journal about everything you did *right* that day.

Day 21

HOW TO LIVE WITH SUGAR

Dear friend, I pray that you may enjoy good health and
that all may go well with you,
even as your soul is getting along well.

—3 John 1:2

Reflect

Throughout this program, you have learned how to live without sugar. Now it's time to reintroduce sugar.

As long as your diet consists primarily of nutrient-dense, whole, low-glycemic foods, you can occasionally enjoy a favorite sweet treat without harming your overall health. When you crave something sweet, choose something nutritious and naturally sweet, such as apples and no-sugar-added nut butter.

However, you may find that avoiding foods high in sugar will only lead you to fixate on "forbidden" foods and want them even more. That's why it's best to take a balanced approach to your diet, including enjoying your favorite treats on occasion. I recommend the 80/20 method—eating 80 percent whole nutritious food, then giving yourself permission to be less-than-perfect 20 percent of the time.

You may feel you don't want sugar anymore, and that's okay. Sugar is a short-term fix for emotional conditions. If you feel your sugar cravings are more than you can handle, take control by reaching out for professional help, either with an experienced psychotherapist specializing in eating disorders and addictions or a registered or licensed dietitian who specializes in behavior and eating disorders for one-on-one support. Another common health concern with excess sugar cravings is candida overgrowth in your intestines. Too much of this yeast in your bowel can drive sugar cravings, make you tired, bloated, irritable, and foggy.

Eating sugar promotes the growth of this intestinal yeast. Having too much yeast in your gut makes you crave more sugar. Candida is naturally present in your intestinal tract. However, if your immune system is weak and your digestion is poor, candida yeast levels can get out of control. Emotional and physical stress can be the main culprit. If you experience this, contact your local integrative health care practitioner or acupuncturist to get tested and treated.

On our last day together, I want to share how I was able to live a life of freedom and balance with sugar.

A few tips for breaking free from the sugar roller coaster.

- Take into consideration how it makes you feel.
- Make sure only to eat a planned treat that you love. Don't settle, and make it memorable. Enjoy it and savor each bite.
- Learn your emotional triggers for overeating or mindless eating.

- Remove foods that trigger you.

- Get an accountability partner, professional counselor, or dietitian to help support you as you learn how to break free.

- Eat well-balanced meals, keep your water bottle nearby, stay well-hydrated, and get the sleep you need.

- Set aside a special day twice a month to enjoy a special treat. Eat it mindfully.

- Know that eating sugar will trigger your desire to eat more. If you find yourself again overwhelmed by sugar cravings, don't panic. You can repeat the 21-Day Sugar Detox. And remember, it only takes about five to seven days to lose the cravings.

- Exercise regularly.

- Find something to do to keep yourself occupied when cravings hit.

Key Points

- It's best to take a balanced approach to your diet, including enjoying your favorite treats on occasion.

- If cravings are more than you can handle, reach out for professional help.

- Candida yeast in your bowel can drive sugar cravings. Get checked for "candida overgrowth" in your intestines.

Put it Into Practice

You have made it to Day 21. Now, decide what is next. I encourage you to stick with your daily plan.

- Wake up with the Lord and rest in His presence when you go to bed at night.

- Talk to him throughout the day, and acknowledge him when you observe nature.
- Thank him when receiving a blessing. Look to him when you need help and a profound yet simple connection.
- Create opportunities to connect with family, loved ones, and good friends.
- Journal your thoughts, breathe, and sip a warm cup of tea.
- Have a weekly date night with your spouse or a fun night with friends.
- Surround yourself with loving, supportive people and turn away from complainers.
- Look for opportunities to serve others who are hurting and struggling and be a blessing to them.
- Continue with the meal plan to continue to stabilize blood sugar levels and sugar cravings.

Prayer

Lord, you are the sweetest and most fulfilling part of my life. I have joy and don't need a poor substitute like sugar to make me happy. Spending time with you fills my need for connection. Thank you for calling me your friend and welcoming me into your arms. Amen.

Affirmation

Write down the following affirmation, take a deep breath, clear any negative thoughts, say it out loud *three* times, and allow it to sink deep into your heart:

> "I turn to the Lord when I am craving connection
> to fulfill all of my needs."

Checkup

Push through to the end of the day. I want to hear you shout HOORAY!

Would you have done anything differently? How did you surprise yourself during this journey?

RECIPES

HOT LEMON WATER

Ingredients

Lemon

2-3 Cups of water

Directions

1. Slice lemons in half and squeeze juice from the slices into a pan with water.

2. Heat water to boiling, then bring it down to a simmer for 5 minutes to allow the lemons to steep in the water.

3. Remove from heat and let it cool for 5 minutes.

4. Add a little cool water if you are short on time and need it to cool more quickly.

5. Pour the water into your mug with one of the lemons from your pan. Doing this will allow the lemon to continue steeping in your water as you drink it.

Nutritional Value

Fat: 0 g, Carbs: 0 g, Protein: 0 g, Total Calories: 0 Calories

APPLE CIDER VINEGAR DETOX RECIPE

Ingredients

1 Cup of Water

2 Tablespoons of Apple Cider Vinegar

2 Tablespoons of Freshly Squeezed Lemon Juice (I like to keep a piece of

lemon in my cup to let steep as I drink it)

1 Dash of Tumeric

1 Teaspoon of Ground Ginger

¼ Teaspoon of Ground Cinnamon

1 Dash of Cayenne Pepper

Directions

1. Combine all of the ingredients into a mug and stir

2. Yes it is spicy. Give it a stir before each sip since the ingredients settle.

3. Reduce the amount of cayenne and gradually increase it up to the amount in the recipe as tolerated.

Nutritional Value

Fat: 0 g, Carbs: 0 g, Protein: 0 g, Total Calories: 0 Calories

GREEN PROTEIN SMOOTHIE

Ingredients

1/2 Frozen Banana

1 Cup of Organic Spinach

1/2 Avocado 1 Serving of Vanilla Protein Powder

1 Cup of Unsweetened Almond Milk

1 Tbsp of Chia Seeds

Directions

1. Start by pouring the almond milk into the blender to avoid the ingredients sticking to the bottom.

2. Add the banana, avocado, spinach, chia seeds, and protein powder.

3. Turn the blender on, starting at a low speed, and increase it as needed.

4. Once the liquid looks smooth, pour it into a cup and enjoy it immediately to conserve as many nutrients as possible.

Nutritional Value

Fat: 20 g, Carbs: 28 g, Protein: 42 g, Total Calories: 430 Calories

ULTIMATE GREEN DETOX JUICE

Ingredients

1 Apple Cut in Half

3 Stalks of Organic Celery, No Leaves

1 Organic Cucumber

8 Organic Kale Leaves

1/2 Lemon Peeled

1 inch of Fresh Ginger

1 Organic Beet

Sprig of mint optional

Directions

1. Wash all the juice ingredients well and pat dry.

2. Cut fruit and vegetables into 1-2 inch chunks. Remove any peels.

3. Place all ingredients in a juicer or blender and strain through a fine mesh strainer to remove fiber or enjoy with fiber.

4. Process into juice according to the manufacturer's directions.

Nutritional Value

Fat: 0 g, Carbs: 0 g, Protein: 0 g, Total Calories: 115 calories

GREEN GINGER CLEANSIING
WEIGHT LOSS JUICE

Ingredients

1 Medium Organic Apple

4 Stalks of Organic Celery

1 Cup of Organic Spinach

1 Organic Cucumber

1 Piece ginger root 1″ diameter

1 Lime peeled

Directions

1. Wash all the ingredients well and pat dry.

2. Cut fruit and vegetables into 1-2 inch chunks.

3. Place all ingredients in a juicer or blender and strain through a fine mesh strainer to remove fiber or enjoy with fiber.

4. Process into juice according to manufacturer's directions.

Nutritional Value

Fat: 0 g, Carbs: 0 g, Protein: 0 g, Total Calories: 195

CHOCOLATE BANANA SMOOTHIE

Ingredients

1 Frozen Banana

1/2 Avocado

1 Cup of Unsweetened Almond Milk (if it is too thick, add a little extra water to ensure the desired consistency is reached)

2 Tbsp of Raw Cacao Powder

1 Serving of Chocolate Protein Powder

Directions

1. Start by pouring the almond milk into the blender to avoid the ingredients sticking to the bottom.

2. Throw in the banana, avocado, cacao powder, and protein powder. Turn the blender on, starting at a low speed, and increase it as needed.

3. Once the liquid looks smooth, pour it into a cup and enjoy it immediately to conserve as many nutrients as possible.

Nutritional Value

Fat: 10 g, Carbs: 54 g, Protein: 41 g, Total Calories: 448 Calories

RASPBERRY COCONUT SMOOTHIE

Ingredients

1 Cup of Organic Raspberries

1/2 Frozen Banana

1 Tbsp of Chia Seeds

1 Cup Unsweetened Coconut Milk

1 Serving of Vanilla Protein Powder

Directions

1. Start by pouring the coconut milk into the blender to avoid the ingredients sticking to the bottom.

2. Add the banana, raspberries, chia seeds, and protein powder.

3. Turn the blender on, starting at a low speed, and increase it as needed.

4. Once the liquid looks smooth, pour it into a cup and enjoy it immediately to conserve as many nutrients as possible.

Nutritional Value

Fat: 10 g Carbs: 54 g Protein: 41 g Total Calories: 448 Calories

BREAKFAST

PALEO BREAKFAST BOWL

Ingredients

2 Eggs

2 oz of Wild caught Smoked Salmon

1/2 Avocado

2 Cups of Sautéed Organic Kale

1 tsp of Olive Oil

1 tsp of Coconut Oil

Directions

1. Start by chopping and washing 2 cups of kale.

2. Once that is done, place a pan on medium heat with a little olive oil and add the kale for about 5 minutes.

3. While the kale is sautéing, prepare the eggs the way you prefer them.

4. Lastly, slice half an avocado and measure 2 oz of smoked salmon.

5. Once everything is ready, combine in a wide bowl and enjoy.

Nutritional Value

Fat: 35 g, Carbs: 20 g, Protein: 29 g, Total Calories: 489 Calories

BANANA PANCAKES

Ingredients

1 Banana

2 Eggs

1 tsp of Ground Cinnamon

1 tsp of Coconut Oil

Directions

1. In a bowl, combine the banana and two eggs.

2. Use a hand blender or a fork to mix the banana and eggs together. Aim for consistency like a pancake batter.

3. Place a pan on medium heat and melt the coconut oil. Slowly add the batter to the pan forming 5-inch diameter pancakes.

4. Place the cover on and cook on each side for a couple of minutes.

5. Repeat until you have cooked the whole batch.

6. Be creative with your toppings, and add any of your favorite clean foods. These may include but are not limited to berries, almond butter, coconut flakes, and chopped nuts.

Nutritional Value

Fat: 24 g, Carbs: 30 g, Protein: 14 g, Total Calories: 378 Calories

MINI OMELETTES

Ingredients

(One Serving)

      3 Eggs

      1/2 Cup of Organic Spinach

      1 Small Organic Tomato

      1 Tbsp of Fresh Basil

      1 Tbsp of Coconut Oil

Directions

1. Preheat the oven to 350F/175C.
2. Coat a muffin tray with coconut oil to avoid sticking.
3. Whisk together the three eggs.
4. Chop the spinach, basil, and tomatoes.
5. Pour the egg mixture into three different muffin cups.
6. Add a bit of the vegetable mixture to each cup, leaving about 1 cm empty at the top.
7. Bake in the oven for 18 minutes.

Nutritional Value

Fat: 29 g, Carbs: 5 g, Protein: 20 g, Total Calories: 360 Calories

BREAKFAST SAUSAGE

Ingredients
(Makes 3 servings)
***1 serving is 2 patties**

    12 oz of Ground Pork

    1 Tbsp of Italian Seasoning

    1/2 Tbsp of Garlic Powder

    1/2 Tbsp of Onion Powder

    1/2 tsp of Sea Salt

    1/4 tsp of Ground Pepper

Directions

1. Combine the pork with all the seasonings in a large bowl.

2. Mix the seasoning into the meat as well as possible and then form 6 patties.

3. Heat a pan on medium heat and add the coconut oil. Once the coconut oil is melted, add all the patties or if you can only fit 4, save a bit of the oil for the second batch.

4. Fry the patties for about 3-5 minutes on each side or until cooked through and browned on the outside.

5. Once they are done, serve immediately warm or store them in a glass container in the fridge for later.

Nutritional Value
(per serving)
Fat: 24 g, Carbs: 0 g, Protein: 19 g, Total Calories: 298 Calories

LUNCH OR DINNER

TUNA SALAD & CUCUMBER

Ingredients

4oz of Tuna

1/2 Avocado

2 Stalks of Celery

1/4 Cup of Red Onions

Pinch of Sea Salt and Pepper

Half of an Organic Cucumber

Directions

1. Drain a can of tuna and pour it into a mixing bowl.
2. Scoop out half of an avocado and mix it with the tuna.
3. Finely chop the celery and red onion and add to the bowl.
4. Season with salt and pepper.
5. Slice half of a cucumber and use the cucumber slices to scoop the tuna salad.

Nutritional Value

Fat: 12 g, Carbs,: 15 g Protein: 33 g, Total Calories: 279 Calories

AVOCADO DEVILED EGGS

Ingredients
(4 Servings)

> 4 Egg
>
> 1/2 Avocado
>
> 1/4 Cup of Mayonnaise
>
> 1 Tbsp of Lime Juice
>
> 1/2 tsp of Salt Pinch of Pepper

Directions

1. Fill a small pot with water up to three-quarters. Bring the water to a boil. Gently add the eggs to the water and boil for 10 minutes.

2. Once the eggs are done, remove them from the pot and add them to a bowl of cold water. Once they have cooled down, peel the shell off.

3. Cut the eggs in half and separate the yolk from the whites.

4. Combine all the yolks in a food processor along with the avocado, mayonnaise, lime juice, salt, and pepper. Process until smooth.

5. Fill the egg white halves with the creamy mixture.

6. Store the deviled eggs in an airtight container in the fridge to avoid browning.

Nutritional Value
(per serving)
Fat: 17 g, Carbs: 3 g, Protein: 7 g, Total Calories: 195 Calories

POWER BOWL

Ingredients

(2 Servings)

4 Cups of Organic Kale

8 oz of Chicken Breast

1 Sweet Potato

1 Avocado

1 Red Bell Pepper

1 tsp Olive Oil

Dressing per Serving:

1 Tbsp of Tahini

1 Tbsp of Lemon Juice

Directions

1. Preheat the oven to 350F/175C. Place the chicken breast and cube-sized sweet potatoes on a baking tray with parchment paper and bake for 30 minutes.

2. Meanwhile, clean and chop the kale. Once the kale is ready, mix it with olive oil and massage it into the kale.

3. Chop the red peppers and avocado.

4. Prepare the dressing by mixing the tahini and fresh lemon juice.

5. Once the chicken and sweet potatoes are done, place the massaged kale at the bottom of a dish and add all the other ingredients on top of it, finishing off with the dressing.

Nutritional Value (per serving)

Fat: 30 g, Carbs: 45 g, Protein: 36 g, Total Calories: 574 Calories

SWEET POTATO SALMON CAKES

Ingredients
(2 Servings)

> 1 Medium Sweet Potato
>
> 8 oz Salmon Filet
>
> 1 Egg
>
> 1/2 Cup of Almond Flour
>
> 1/4 Cup of Green Onions
>
> 1 tsp of Sea Salt
>
> 1/4 tsp of Black Pepper

Directions

1. Preheat the oven to 400F/200C and line a baking sheet with parchment paper.
2. Wash and peel te sweet potato and steam until soft.
3. Bake the salmon for about 15-20 minutes.
4. Once the sweet potato is soft and the salmon is cooked, mash them together in a bowl.
5. Place the remaining ingredients in the bowl.
6. Form 8 patties and spread them out on the baking sheet.
7. Bake the Sweet Potato Salmon cakes for 30 minutes; flip the patties at around 15 minutes.
8. Serve on its own or with a green salad.

Nutritional Value
(per serving)
Fat: 25 g, Carbs: 25 g, Protein: 30 g, Total Calories: 434 Calories

BEEF FAJITA BOWL

Ingredients (2 Servings)

- 8oz Beef Strips
- 1 Organic Red Bell Pepper
- 1/2 Cup of Onions
- 2 Cloves of Garlic
- 1/2 Cup of Brown Rice
- 1 Avocado
- 1 Tbsp of Coconut Oil

Fajita Seasoning:

- 1 Tbsp Paprika
- 1 tsp Garlic Powder
- 1 tsp Onion Powder
- 1/2 tsp Cayenne Powder

Directions

1. Prepare the rice according to the package directions.
2. Place a pan on medium heat and add the coconut oil. Once the oil has melted, add the onions, and garlic, and sauté for 1 minute.
3. Add the beef strips and cook for 3-5 minutes.
4. Meanwhile, cut the red pepper into strips. Once the beef is ready, add the peppers and all the fajita seasoning spices and cook for 5 minutes.
5. Combine in a bowl the beef mixture, brown rice and mashed avocado.

Nutritional Value (per serving)

Fat: 10 g, Carbs: 41 g, Protein: 27 g, Total Calories: 330 Calories

CHICKEN COBB SALAD

Ingredients
(2 Servings)

> 4 Cups of Organic Spinach
>
> 8 oz of Chicken
>
> 2 Hard Boiled Egg
>
> 4 Slices of No Sugar Uncured Bacon
>
> 1 Cup of Chopped Organic Cucumber
>
> 1 Avocado
>
> 2 Tbsp of Extra Virgin Olive Oil
>
> 1 Pinch of Sea Salt and Pepper

Directions

1. Preheat the oven to 350F/175C.
2. Bake the chicken breast in a dish with olive oil, salt , and pepper for about 30 minutes.
3. While the chicken is cooking, wash the spinach and place it at the base of a salad bowl.
4. Place all the remaining ingredients on top of the spinach.
5. Once the chicken is done, add it to the bowl.
6. Lastly drizzle the olive oil on top and add sea salt and pepper, if desired.

Nutritional Value
(per serving)
Fat: 39 g, Carbs: 10 g, Protein: 39 g, Total Calories: 524 Calories

PALEO SUSHI BOWL

Ingredients

1 Sheet of Nori

2 Cups of Cauliflower Rice

3.5 oz of Smoked Wild Caught Salmon

1/2 Avocado

2 Tbsp of Coconut Aminos

Directions

1. Start with making the cauliflower rice by grating cauliflower.

2. Scoop out half of an avocado.

3. Combine everything in a large bowl, with the cauliflower being the base.

4. Next, add in either raw sushi-grade salmon or you can also use smoked salmon.

5. Finally, add one sheet of nori seaweed cut into small strips and top it all off with some coconut aminos.

Nutritional Value

Fat: 27 g, Carbs: 21 g, Protein: 28 g, Total Calories: 403 Calories

BAKED SALMON

Ingredients

4 oz of Wild Caught Salmon Fillet

1/4 Cup of Brown Rice

10 Stalks of Asparagus

1 Tbsp of Olive Oil

Directions

1. Start by pre-heating the oven at 350F/175C.

2. Cut off the ends of the asparagus and wash it. Coat the salmon and asparagus with olive oil, salt, and pepper. Line a baking tray with parchment paper, add the salmon and asparagus to the baking tray, and bake for 20 minutes.

3. Meanwhile, prepare the rice by adding 1/2 cup of water and the rice to a pot. Bring to a boil, then turn the heat down to a simmer until all the water is absorbed.

4. Plate the salmon, asparagus, and brown rice together and enjoy.

Nutritional Value

Fat: 22 g, Carbs: 29 g, Protein: 28 g, Total Calories: 419 Calories

CHICKEN CURRY

Ingredients

(Makes 2 Servings)

> 8 oz of Chicken
>
> 2 Cup of Organic Broccoli
>
> 1 Carrot Sliced
>
> 1/2 Cup of Chopped Onions
>
> 1 Can of Unsweetened Coconut Milk
>
> 2 Cups of Cauliflower Rice
>
> 1 Tbsp of Ground Turmeric
>
> 1 Tbsp of Ground Cumin
>
> 1 Tbsp of Ground Ginger

Directions

1. Place a pan on medium heat and melt one teaspoon of coconut oil.

2. Place the chicken in the pan and cook until it is well done.

3. Take the chicken out of the pan and set aside. Add another teaspoon of the coconut oil and all the vegetables and spices to the pan.

4. Let the vegetables sauté for 5 minutes, add the coconut milk, and cook for another 5 minutes.

5. Lastly, add the chicken back in and mix well. Serve on top of cauliflower rice.

Nutritional Value

(1 Serving)

Fat: 35 g, Carbs: 18 g, Protein: 35 g, Total Calories: 350 Calories

TOMATO & GARLIC SPAGHETTI SQUASH

Ingredients (2 Servings)

1 Small Spaghetti Squash

8 oz of Chicken Breast

1 Can of Diced Tomatoes

2 Cloves of Garlic

1/4 Cup of Onions

2 Tbsp of Extra Virgin Olive Oil

Directions

1. Start by preheating the oven to 400F/200C.

2. Cut your spaghetti squash into two halves and take the seeds out with a spoon.

3. Bake the squash with the peel on the bottom of a baking tray for 45 minutes.

4. While the squash is cooking, you can prepare the sauce by placing a pan on low-medium heat and adding olive oil.

5. Next, add the garlic, onion, and diced tomatoes.

6. Slice the chicken breasts and add them to the pan. Stir every few minutes to make sure the chicken cooks evenly.

7. Once the garlic and tomato sauce is ready, you can set it aside on low heat and wait for the squash to be done.

8. After 45 minutes, take the squash out and use a fork to scrape out the squash into spaghetti-like strings.

9. Top it off with the chicken garlic tomato sauce.

Nutritional Value (per serving)
Fat: 38 g, Carbs: 33 g, Protein: 27 g, Total Calories: 557 Calories

VEGGIE SCRAMBLE & AVOCADO

Ingredients

2 Eggs

1 Cup of Organic Spinach

2 Mushrooms

1/4 Organic Red Bell Pepper

1/4 Cup of Red Onions

1/2 Avocado

1 tsp of Coconut Oil

Directions

1. Heat a pan on medium heat and add the coconut oil. Once the coconut oil is melted, add all the vegetables except for the spinach and cook for 3 minutes.

2. Next add the eggs and spinach.

3. Once the omelet is complete add the sliced avocado on top.
   4. Season with salt and pepper to your desire.

Nutritional Value

Fat: 39 g,Carbs: 16 g, Protein: 16g, Total Calories: 460 Calories

SHRIMP PAD THAI

Ingredients

(2 Servings)

2 Organic Zucchinis

8 oz of Shrimp

1 Cup of Bean Sprouts

1 Clove of Garlic 1/2 Cup Green Onions

1/4 Cup of Coconut Aminos

2 Tbsp of Unsweetened Almond Butter

1 Tbsp of Coconut Oil

Directions

1. Place a pan on medium heat and add the coconut oil.

2. Finely chop the garlic and add it to the pan with the shrimps.

3. When the shrimps are ready add in the bean sprouts.

4. Mix the coconut aminos and the almond butter to form a thick sauce and toss it in the pan and lower the heat.

5. Meanwhile spiralize the zucchini and add it in the pan for the last 3 minutes to let it warm up a little bit but don't leave the zucchini noodles in for too long or else they will become overly soft.

Nutritional Value

(per serving)

Fat: 17 g, Carbs: 31 g, Protein: 39 g, Tot al Calories: 407 Calories

CHICKEN AVOCADO SALAD

Ingredients
(2 Servings)

8 oz of Chicken Breast

2 Organic Tomatoes

1 Cup Diced Organic Cucumber

1 Avocado 1/2 Cup of Red Onions

1 Tbsp of Olive Oil Pinch of Sea Salt and Pepper

Directions

1. Preheat the oven to 350F/175C.

2. In the oven, place the chicken breast in a dish with olive oil and cover for about 30 minutes.

3. While the chicken is cooking, chop the cucumber, tomatoes, red onion, and avocado into small cubes.

4. Combine all the vegetables in a large bowl. Once the chicken is cooked, let it cool down and shred it with a fork.

5. Add the chicken to the vegetables. Mix with the avocado oil, salt and pepper to finish.

Nutritional Value
(per serving)
Fat: 27 g, Carbs: 16 g, Protein: 27 g, Total Calories: 406 Calories

ZUCCHINI NOODLES & BOLOGNESE

Ingredients (2 Servings)

> 2 Organic Zucchinis
>
> 16 oz of Ground Beef
>
> 1/2 Cup of Unsweetened Coconut Milk
>
> 1/4 Cup of Tomato Paste 1 Cup of Organic Spinach
>
> 1 Organic Carrot 6 Mushrooms
>
> 1/2 Cup of Onions
>
> 2 Cloves of Garlic
>
> 1 Tbsp of Coconut Oil

Directions

1. Chop the onions, garlic, and mushrooms.
2. In a pan melt the coconut oil and add the onions and garlic, once the onions become translucent add in the ground beef and season with salt and pepper.
3. Once the ground beef is cooked through, add the chopped mushrooms and spinach. In a small bowl combine the coconut milk and tomato paste and mix until it forms a thick sauce.
4. Add the coconut milk and tomato paste mixture to the skillet and turn the heat down to low, let simmer for about 10 minutes.
5. While the Bolognese is cooking wash 1 zucchini and spiralize it into noodles.
6. Serve the Bolognese on top of the spiralized zucchini.

Nutritional Value
(per serving)
Fat: 25 g, Carbs: 10 g, Protein: 28 g, Total Calories: 374 Calories

CHICKEN ALMOND BUTTER STIR FRY

Ingredients
(2 Servings)

> 8 oz Chicken Breast
>
> 2 Cups Organic Broccoli
>
> 1 Organic Red Bell Pepper
>
> 4 Mushrooms
>
> 1/2 Cup of Red Onions
>
> 1/4 Cup of Coconut Aminos
>
> 2 Tbsp of Unsweetened Almond Butter
>
> 1 Tbsp of Coconut Oil

Directions

1. Chop all the vegetables into bite-size pieces.
2. Place a pan on medium heat and melt the coconut oil.
3. Slice the chicken and add to the pan.
4. Meanwhile, combine the coconut aminos and almond butter and whisk until it forms a thick sauce.
5. Once the chicken in cooked, add all the vegetables and the almond butter sauce.
6. Cook and cover for another 7-10 minutes.
7. Turn the heat off, remove the cover, and let the sauce thicken up for a few minutes before serving.

Nutritional Value
(per serving)
Fat: 35 g, Carbs: 53 g, Protein: 32 g, Total Calories: 534 Calories

TURKEY LETTUCE BURGERS

Ingredients
(2 Servings)

16 oz of Ground Turkey

1 Cup of Organic Spinach

1/4 Cup of Onions

1 Clove of Garlic

1 Tbsp of Coconut Oil

Directions

1. Chop the spinach, onions, and garlic in a mixing bowl with the ground turkey, salt and pepper.
2. Melt the coconut oil on medium heat in a pan.
3. Form 6 patties and fry each side for 3-5 minutee.
4. Once the burgers are ready add your favorite toppings on top of the patties and enjoy.

Nutritional Value
(per serving)
Fat: 25 g, Carbs: 3 g, Protein: 40 g, Total Calories: 405 Calories

SCHNITZEL & SWEET POTATO FRIES

Ingredients (2 Servings)

8 oz of Thin Turkey Breast

1/2 Cup of Almond Flour

1 Egg 1 tsp of Garlic Powder

1 tsp of Onion Powder

1 Medium Sweet Potato

1 Tbsp of Olive Oil

1 tsp of Sea Salt

1/2 tsp of Ground Pepper

Directions

1. Preheat the oven to 400F/200C. While the oven is pre-heating, wash, peel and cut the sweet potato into the shape of fries. Toss them in a bowl with the olive oil, salt, and pepper, and then line them up on a baking sheet lined with parchment paper. Bake in the oven for 30 minutes.

2. Place a pan on medium heat and melt the coconut oil. Start preparing the schnitzels by combining the almond flour and spices in one bowl and whisking the egg in another. Dip the turkey slice into the egg mixture and the almond flour, ensuring you cover as much meat as possible.

3. Place the coated schnitzel in the pan and cook until both sides are golden, and the meat is cooked well.

Nutritional Value
(per serving)
Fat: 23 g, Carbs: 40 g, Protein: 46 g, Total Calories: 546 Calories

BEEF & BROCCOLI

Ingredients

(2 Servings)

8 oz Beef Strips

2 Cups of Organic Broccoli

1/2 Cup of Brown Rice

1/4 Cup of Coconut Aminos

1/2 Cup of Onions

1 Cloves of Garlic

1 Tbsp of Coconut Oil

Directions

1. Start by bringing 1 cup of water with the rice to a boil. Once the water is boiling, bring it down to a simmer.

2. Next, finely chop the onion and garlic. Place a large pan on medium heat and add the coconut oil. Once the oil has melted, add the onions and garlic.

3. Once the onions are translucent, add the beef strips to the pan and cook for 3-5 minutes.

4. Cut the broccoli into small florets and add them to the pan along with the coconut aminos.

5. Cover and cook on low heat for 10 minutes. Once the beef and broccoli are done, serve them on top of the brown rice.

Nutritional Value

Fat: 23 g, Carbs: 52 g, Protein: 28 g, Total Calories: 454 Calories

SNACKS & TREATS

CARROTS & ALMOND BUTTER

Ingredients

> 2 Organic Carrots
>
> 1 Tbsp of Almond Butter

Directions

Slice the carrots into sticks and use the almond butter as a dip.

Nutritional Value

Fat: 19 g ,Carbs: 13 g, Protein: 5 g, Total Calories: 229 Calories

ALMOND BUTTER FUDGES

Ingredients (Makes 6)

- 1/4 Cup of Coconut Oil
- 1/4 Cup of Unsweetened Almond Butter
- 1/4 Cup of Raw Cacao Powder

Directions

1. Start by melting the coconut oil and then add the almond butter and the cacao powder to the melted coconut oil.
2. Mix until it forms a smooth mixture.
3. Add 2 Tbsp of the mixture in silicon muffin cups.
4. Freeze the fudge for an hour before consuming. Keep them stored in the freezer.

Nutritional Value

Fat: 31 g, Carbs: 8 g, Net Carbs: 4 g, Protein: 7 g Total Calories: 300 Calories

EASY TRAIL MIX

Ingredients

(3 servings)

> 1/2 Cup of Unsweetened Coconut Chips
>
> 1/4 Cup of Almonds
>
> 1/4 Cup of Pumpkin Seeds

Directions

1. Place all the ingredients in an airtight jar and store somewhere cool or immediately divide the trail mix into 3 portions.

Nutritional Value

(per serving)

Fat: 20 g, Carbs: 9 g, Protein: 10 g, Total Calories: 256 Calories

COCONUT CHIA PUDDING

Ingredients
(4 Servings)

> 1 Can of Coconut Milk
>
> 1/4 Cup of Chia Seeds
>
> 1/4 Cup of Organic Berries
>
> 1 tsp of Vanilla Extract

Directions

1. Combine all the ingredients in a bowl except the berries. Stir well and then transfer the mixture to a sealed container.

2. Let the chia seed pudding sit in the refrigerator for 3 hours or overnight.

3. Once it is ready, you can separate it into four servings and add a handful of berries.

Nutritional Value
(per serving)
Fat: 25 g, Carbs: 11 g, Net Carbs: 3 g, Protein: 5 g, Total Calories: 286 Calories

SIMPLE MILLS ORGANIC SEED CRACKERS & GUACAMOLE

Ingredients
(Makes 3 Servings)
27 Simple Mills Organic Seed Crackers
Guacamole: 1/2 Mashed Avocado Juice of Half a Lime optional chopped red bell pepper and cliantro

Directions

1. Combine the guacamole ingredients in a bowl and mash until you have your desired consistency.

2. Garnish Simple Mills crackers with guacamole.

Nutritional Value
(per serving)
Fat: 12g, Carbs: 18 g, Protein: 2.57g, Total Calories: 195 Calories

PAY IT FORWARD

Thank you from the bottom of my heart for reading my book. I put all of myself into this body of work and pray that it blesses you. If it has made a difference in your life, there's a simple way to pay it forward. Just take a few minutes to share your testimony, to point the way for others who are searching for the freedom you've found.

Visit this link, which will take you directly to Amazon: Review.21DaysWithoutSugar.com

I appreciate it so much and promise to read your review!

ACKNOWLEDGMENTS

I must start by thanking my loving and supportive husband, Corey. In supporting me, he does his best to keep up with my ever-changing passionate ideas and believes in me.

He was as essential to getting this book completed as I was. Thank you, Corey, for taking care of preparing dinners, getting the kids to bed, and getting the dishes done so I could write and edit. Your loving support means everything.

To my Father God for putting the desire in me to inspire and educate others from my overflowing passion. His love, support, and reminders in the middle of the night and early mornings of who I am and what my mission is kept me going.

To my children, Cooper, Camble, and Charlotte, for keeping me on my toes and remaining patient when I wasn't available or my brain was too tired. I am thankful to be your teacher, which keeps me excited about learning and teaching.

To Donna Partow for coaching me on the journey to creating my first book. For believing in me and my message for the world. I am grateful for your encouragement and deadlines to continue on the path of excellence as the only option.

To my lovely, talented, and super intelligent friends Shannon Chance, Teresa Stowe, Diane Minkner, HHP, BIT, AK, QRT, for taking the time to review this book with a critical eye to make it perfect. Thank you, ladies. I am grateful to have you in my life.

ABOUT THE AUTHOR

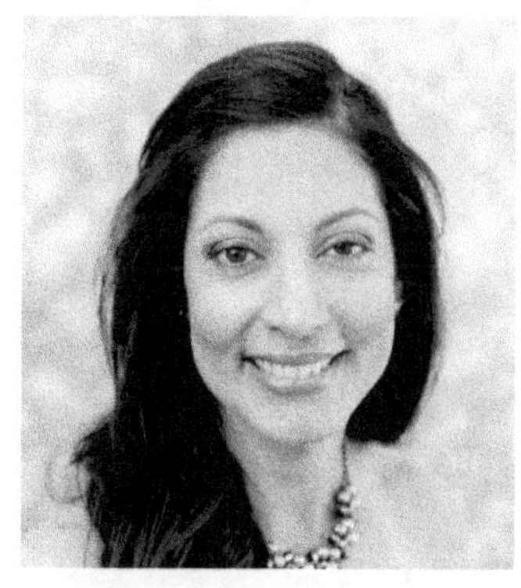

I am a homeschooling mom of three and married to my supportive husband, Corey. I love to exercise and need it daily for my sanity. I am thankful for my family and the freedom to live where we want.

I am a registered dietitian and licensed dietitian. I am a fitness specialist with more than twenty-two years experience treating clients in private practice and virtual programs and courses. Along with treating clinical conditions, I specialize in helping clients achieve their best health and enjoy a peaceful relationship with food and balanced eating.

I am passionate about learning, sharing, supporting, and educating the community to better physical, emotional, and spiritual health.

GET EXTRA SUPPORT

For extra support on your detox journey, join my Sugar Detox group. In this group, you will learn from other women who share in your journey and are ready to give you the support you need. You may also find that others in the group need your wisdom and encouragement.

This is for you if you struggle with sugar and need a fresh start and group support.

Grab your spot in my Sugar Detox Online group. You will receive daily education, inspiration and coaching, and support from me and others on the same sugar-free journey.

Visit the link below to learn more:

www.21dayswithoutsugar.com

WELL WITHIN LIFESTYLE ACADEMY

Balance your hormones,
end bad eating habits, and lose weight.

The program includes three individual private sessions with me, valued at $360.

Learn More Here:

www.wellwithinutrition.com/well-within-lifestyle-academy

This program is for you if you:

Struggle to lose weight and keep it off despite everything you have tried.

Struggle with anxiety and a love/hate relationship with food.

Self-sabotage when embarking on a new weight loss program and finding yourself bitter and angry.

This online course:

- Is self-paced.
- Includes comprehensive with full online easy access.
- Combines thoughts, behaviors, nutrition, and fitness.
- Teaches how to lose weight and maintain your health without ever starting another diet again.
- Includes monthly online group coaching, accountability, and support led by Cynthia Ray.